HIGH-YIELD™

FIFTH EDITION | Neuroanatomy

Douglas J. Gould, PhD
Professor and Vice Chair
Department of Biomedical Sciences
William Beaumont School of Medicine
Oakland University
Rochester, Michigan

Jennifer K. Brueckner-Collins, PhD
Professor and Vice Chair
Department of Anatomical Sciences and Neurobiology
University of Louisville School of Medicine
Louisville, Kentucky

Author of First-Fourth Editions:
James D. Fix, PhD
(1931–2010)

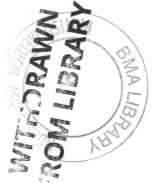
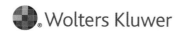
. Wolters Kluwer

Philadelphia • Baltimore • New York • London
Buenos Aires • Hong Kong • Sydney • Tokyo

Acquisitions Editor: Crystal Taylor
Product Development Editor: Stephanie Roulias
Director of Medical Marketing: Lisa Zoks
Production Project Manager: Bridgett Dougherty
Design Coordinator: Teresa Mallon
Manufacturing Coordinator: Margie Orzech
Prepress Vendor: Aptara, Inc.

Fifth edition

9 8 7 6 5 4 3 2 1

Printed in China

978-1-4511-9343-5
Library of Congress Cataloging-in-Publication Data
available upon request

I dedicate this work to my beloved wife, Marie. Your strength, courage, and love are the engine that moves our family forward and provides the foundation for our girls to grow into proud, strong women. I love you. Thank you.

Douglas J. Gould

I dedicate my contributions to this book to my son, Lincoln. You are the light of my life and you make each and every day meaningful and fun! You have already taught me a lifetime of lessons about love, life, and the importance of play in the short 9 1/2 months that we have had together and I am eternally grateful to you for that. I hope that we will have the blessed opportunity to share many more years learning from and loving each other. I love you to the moon and back, my sweet bunny.

Jennifer K. Brueckner-Collins

Based on your feedback on previous editions of this text, the fifth edition has been reorganized and updated significantly in order to provide an accurate and quick review of important clinical aspects of neuroanatomy for the future physician. New features include the replacement of the "key concepts" with more focused "objectives" for each chapter, driving the content, order, and level of detail. The chapters have been reordered and recombined to group "like" topic more closely. A new *Gross Structure* chapter has been incorporated to lay the foundation for understanding the sectional anatomy in the *Atlas* chapter. The fourth edition's *Thalamus* and *Hypothalamus* chapters are now integrated in the fifth edition as a new *Diencephalon* chapter; the previous *Spinal cord*, *Spinal cord tracts*, and *Spinal cord lesions* chapters are combined in a centralized *Spinal Cord* chapter; and the former *Brainstem* and *Brainstem lesions* chapters are united in a new *Brainstem* chapter. Terminology updates have been included to ensure consistency with *Terminologica Anatomica.*

We would appreciate receiving your comments and/or suggestions concerning *High-Yield™ Neuroanatomy* Fifth Edition especially after you have taken the USMLE Step 1 examination. Your suggestions will find their way into the sixth edition. You may contact us at djgould@oakland.edu or jkbrue02@louisville.edu.

CONTENTS

CHAPTER 1

Gross Structure of the Brain

Objectives

1. Describe the telencephalon including the lobes of the cerebral hemispheres and the major gyri, sulci and lobules of each.
2. Differentiate the structures of the limbic and olfactory senses from other parts of the brain.
3. List the different parts of the diencephalon, brainstem, and cerebellum.

I **Divisions of the Brain.** The brain consists of five divisions: **telencephalon, diencephalon, mesencephalon, metencephalon, and myelencephalon.**

A. Telencephalon consists of the **cerebral hemispheres** and the **basal nuclei.** The cerebral hemispheres contain the **lateral ventricles.**

1. **Cerebral hemispheres (Figures 1-1 to 1-3)** consist of six lobes and the olfactory structures:

   a. **Frontal lobe** extends from the central sulcus to the frontal pole and lies superior to the lateral sulcus. It contains:
      - **Precentral gyrus**—consists of the primary motor area (area 4).
      - **Superior frontal gyrus**—contains supplementary motor cortex on the medial surface (area 6).
      - **Middle frontal gyrus**—contains the frontal eye field (area 8).
      - **Inferior frontal gyrus**—contains the Broca speech area in the dominant hemisphere (areas 44 and 45).
      - **Gyrus rectus and orbital gyri**—separated by the olfactory sulcus.
      - **Anterior paracentral lobule**—found on the medial surface between the superior frontal gyrus (paracentral sulcus) and the central sulcus.

   b. **Parietal lobe** extends from the central sulcus to the occipital lobe and lies superior to the temporal lobe.
      - **Postcentral gyrus**—the primary somatosensory area of the cerebral cortex (areas 3, 1, and 2).
      - **Superior parietal lobule** comprises association areas involved in somatosensory functions (areas 5 and 7).
      - **Inferior parietal lobule** consists of the **supramarginal gyrus,** which interrelates somatosensory, auditory, and visual inputs (area 40) and the **angular gyrus** (area 39) that receives impulses from primary visual cortex.
      - **Precuneus**—located between the paracentral lobule and the cuneus.
      - **Posterior paracentral lobule**—located on the medial surface between the central sulcus and the precuneus.

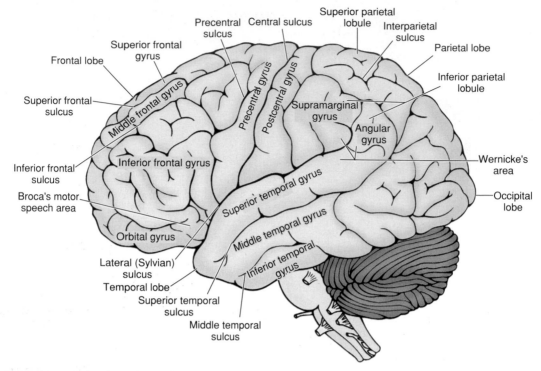

Figure 1-1 Lateral surface of the brain showing the principal gyri and sulci.

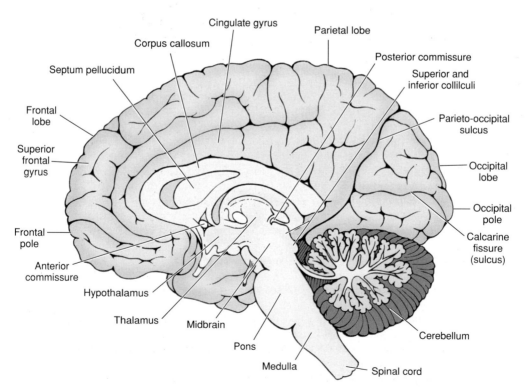

Figure 1-2 Midsagittal section of the brain and brainstem showing the structures surrounding the third and fourth ventricles.

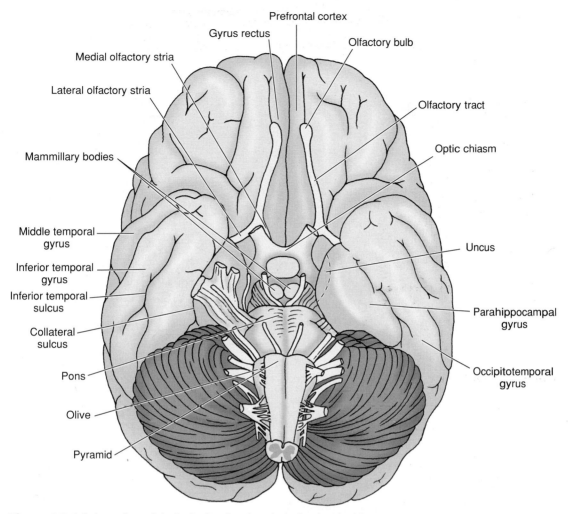

Figure 1-3 Inferior surface of the brain showing the principal gyri and sulci.

c. **Temporal lobe** extends from the temporal pole to the occipital lobe, inferior to the lateral sulcus. It contains:
- **Transverse temporal gyrus (of Heschl)**—found within the lateral sulcus. It contains the primary auditory areas of the cerebral cortex (areas 41 and 42).
- **Superior temporal gyrus**—associated with auditory functions and contains the **Wernicke speech area** in the dominant hemisphere (area 22).
- **Middle temporal gyrus**
- **Inferior temporal gyrus**
- **Lateral occipitotemporal gyrus (fusiform gyrus)**—lies between the inferior temporal sulcus and the collateral sulcus.

d. **Occipital lobe** lies posterior to a line connecting the parieto-occipital sulcus and the preoccipital notch. It contains two structures:
- **Cuneus**—situated between the parieto-occipital sulcus and the calcarine sulcus and contains the visual cortex (areas 17, 18, and 19).
- **Lingual gyrus** lies inferior to the calcarine sulcus and contains the visual cortex (areas 17, 18, and 19).

e. **Insular lobe** (insula) lies within the lateral sulcus.

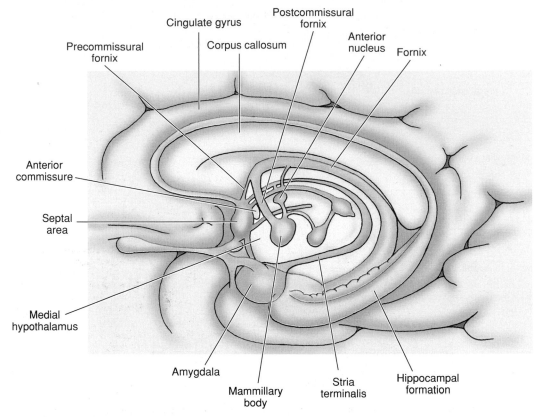

Figure 1-4 Midsagittal section of the brain showing the components of the limbic lobe.

    f. Limbic lobe (Figure 1-4)—a C-shaped collection of structures found on the medial hemispheric surface that encircles the corpus callosum and the lateral aspect of the midbrain. It includes:
- **Paraterminal gyrus and subcallosal area**—located anterior to the lamina terminalis and inferior to the rostrum of the corpus callosum.
- **Cingulate gyrus** lies parallel and superior to the corpus callosum and merges with the parahippocampal gyrus.
- **Parahippocampal gyrus** lies between the hippocampal and collateral sulci and terminates in the **uncus.**
- **Hippocampal formation** (Figure 1-5)—connected to the hypothalamus and septal area via the **fornix.**

    g. Olfactory structures—found on the orbital (inferior) surface of the brain and include the following:
- **Olfactory bulb and tract** represent an outpouching of the telencephalon. The olfactory bulb receives the olfactory nerve (CN I).
- **Olfactory trigone and striae**
- **Anterior perforated substance** created by penetrating striate arteries.
- **Diagonal band of Broca** interconnects the amygdaloid nucleus and the septal area.

  2. Basal nuclei (ganglia) (Figure 1-6) constitute the subcortical nuclei of the telencephalon and include:
    a. Caudate nucleus—part of the striatum, together with the putamen.
    b. Putamen—part of the striatum, together with the caudate nucleus and part of the lentiform nucleus along with the globus pallidus.
    c. Globus pallidus—part of the lentiform nucleus, together with the putamen.
    d. Subthalamic nucleus—part of the diencephalon that functions with the basal nuclei.

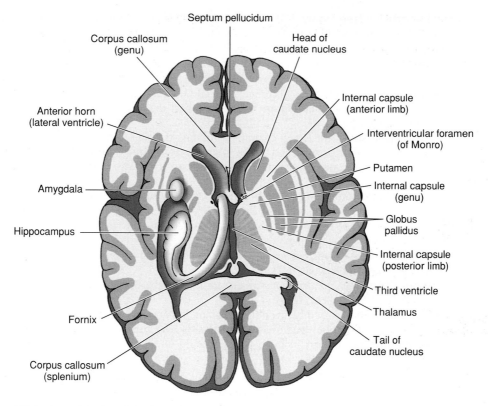

Figure 1-5 Horizontal section of the brain showing the components of the internal capsule.

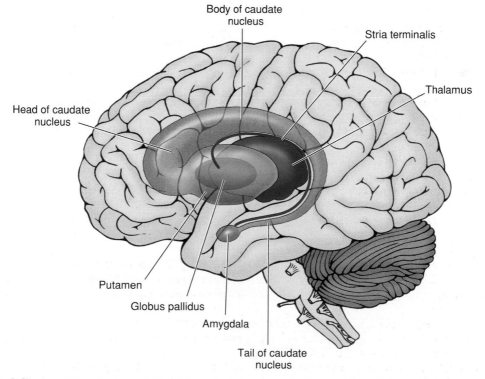

Figure 1-6 Schematic diagram of basal nuclei.

3. **Lateral ventricles (see Figure 1-5)**—ependyma-lined cavities of the cerebral hemispheres that contain **CSF** and **choroid plexus.** They communicate with the third ventricle via two interventricular foramina (of Monro) and are separated from each other by the septum pellucidum.
4. **Cerebral cortex** consists of a thin layer or mantle of gray matter that covers the surface of each cerebral hemisphere and is folded into gyri that are separated by sulci.
5. **White matter** includes the cerebral commissures and the internal capsule.
   a. **Cerebral commissures (see Figure 1-2)** interconnect the cerebral hemispheres and include the following structures:
      - **Corpus callosum**—the largest commissure of the brain and it interconnects the two hemispheres. It has four parts, including the **rostrum, genu, body, and splenium.**
      - **Anterior commissure**—interconnects the olfactory bulbs with the middle and inferior temporal lobes.
      - **Hippocampal commissure (commissure of the fornix)**—located between the fornices and inferior to the splenium of the corpus callosum.
   b. **Internal capsule (see Figure 1-5)** consists of the white matter located between the basal nuclei and the thalamus. It has five parts:
      - **Anterior limb**—located between the caudate nucleus and putamen and contains a mixture of ascending and descending fibers.
      - **Genu**—located between the anterior and posterior limbs and contains primarily the corticonuclear (corticobulbar) fibers.
      - **Posterior limb**—located between the thalamus and lentiform nucleus (comprising the putamen and the globus pallidus) and is primarily made up of corticospinal fibers.
      - **Retrolenticular portion**—located posterior to the lentiform nucleus and contains the optic radiations.

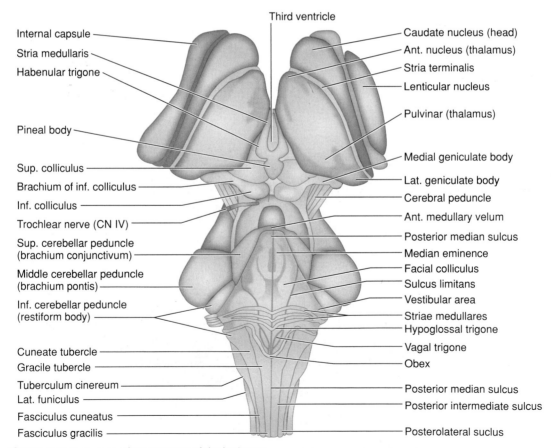

Figure 1-7 Posterior surface anatomy of the brainstem.

- **Sublenticular portion**—located inferior to the lentiform nucleus and contains auditory radiations.

B. Diencephalon (see Figures 1-2 and 1-7) receives the optic nerve (CN II) and consists of the following structures:
1. **Epithalamus**
2. **(Dorsal) Thalamus**—separated from the hypothalamus by the **hypothalamic sulcus.**
3. **Hypothalamus** (Figure 1-8)
4. **Subthalamus (ventral thalamus)**—inferior to the thalamus and lateral to the hypothalamus.
5. **Third ventricle and associated structures.**

C. Mesencephalon (Midbrain) (see Figures 1-7 and 1-8)—located between the diencephalon and the pons and contains the **cerebral aqueduct** interconnecting the third and fourth ventricles.
1. **Anterior surface**
   a. **Cerebral peduncle**
   b. **Interpeduncular fossa**
      i. *Oculomotor nerve (CN III)*
      ii. *Posterior perforated substance*—created by the penetrating branches of the posterior cerebral and posterior communicating arteries.
2. **Posterior surface**
   a. **Superior colliculus (visual system)**
   b. **Brachium of the superior colliculus**

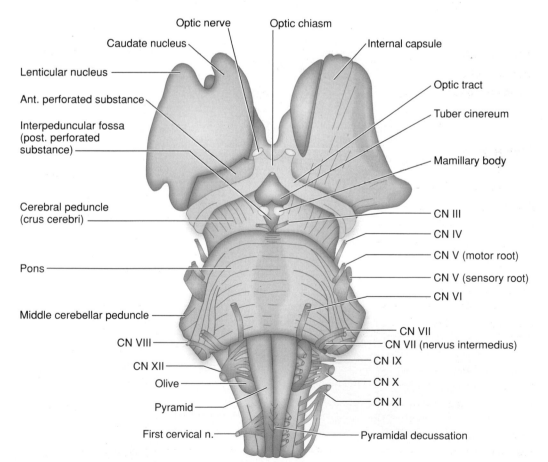

Figure 1-8 Anterior surface anatomy of the brainstem.

    c. Inferior colliculus (auditory system)
    d. Brachium of the inferior colliculus
    e. Trochlear nerve (CN IV)—the only cranial nerve to exit the brainstem from the posterior aspect.

D. Pons (see Figures 1-7 and 1-8)—located between the midbrain and the medulla.
    1. Anterior surface
        a. Base of the pons
        b. Cranial nerves, including trigeminal nerve (CN V), abducent nerve (CN VI), facial nerve (CN VII), and vestibulocochlear nerve (CN VIII)
    2. Posterior surface (rhomboid fossa)
        a. Locus ceruleus contains the largest collection of norepinephrinergic neurons in the CNS.
        b. Facial colliculus contains the abducent nucleus and internal genu of the facial nerve.
        c. Sulcus limitans separates the alar plate from the basal plate.
        d. Striae medullares of the rhomboid fossa divides the rhomboid fossa into the superior pontine portion and the inferior medullary portion.

E. Medulla Oblongata (myelencephalon) (see Figures 1-7 and 1-8)—located between the pons and the spinal cord.
    1. Anterior surface
        a. Pyramid contains descending tracts.
        b. Olive contains the inferior olivary nucleus.

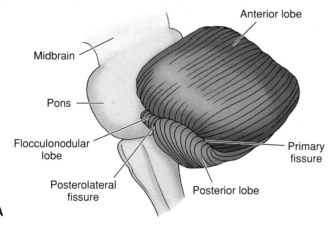

A

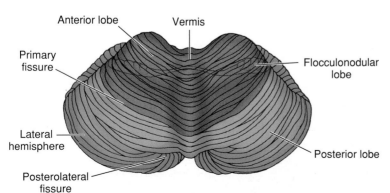

B

Figure 1-9 Surface features of the cerebellum from a lateral view **(A)** and a posterior view **(B).**

      c. **Cranial nerves,** including glossopharyngeal nerve (CN IX), vagus nerve (CN X), (spinal) accessory nerve (CN XI), and hypoglossal nerve (CN XII)

  2. Posterior surface
      a. Gracile tubercle
      b. Cuneate tubercle
      c. Rhomboid fossa
         i. Striae medullares of the rhomboid fossa
         ii. Vagal trigone
         iii. Hypoglossal trigone
         iv. Sulcus limitans
         v. Area postrema (vomiting center)

F. Cerebellum (Figures 1-7 and 1-9)—located in the posterior cranial fossa, attached to the brainstem by three cerebellar peduncles. It forms the roof of the fourth ventricle. It is separated from the occipital and temporal lobes by the **tentorium cerebelli** and contains the following surface structures/parts:

  1. Hemispheres consist of two lateral lobes.
  2. Vermis
  3. Flocculus and vermal nodulus form the flocculonodular lobule.
  4. Tonsil is a rounded lobule on the inferior surface of each cerebellar hemisphere. With increased intracranial pressure, it may herniate through the foramen magnum.
  5. Superior cerebellar peduncle connects the cerebellum to the pons and midbrain.
  6. Middle cerebellar peduncle connects the cerebellum to the pons.
  7. Inferior cerebellar peduncle connects the cerebellum to the pons and medulla.
  8. Anterior lobe lies anterior to the primary fissure.
  9. Posterior lobe is located between the primary and posterolateral fissures.
 10. Flocculonodular lobe lies posterior to the posterolateral fissure.

CHAPTER 2

Development of the Nervous System

Objectives

1. Describe the development of the neural tube, including the stages of development and the adult derivatives of each brain vesicle.
2. Trace the lineage of the cells of the neural tube wall, including the alar and basal plates.
3. Identify the derivatives of the neural crest.
4. Describe the development of the brainstem as well as the general arrangement of motor versus sensory components and somatic versus visceral components.
5. Describe the development of the pituitary (hypophysis).
6. List and characterize major congenital malformations of the central nervous system.

 I **The Neural Tube** (Figure 2-1) gives rise to the **central nervous system (CNS)** (i.e., brain and spinal cord).

A. The **brainstem** and spinal cord are composed of plates separated by the sulcus limitans:
   1. An **alar plate**—gives rise to **sensory neurons.**
   2. A **basal plate**—gives rise to **motor neurons** (Figure 2-2).
   3. **Interneurons** are derived from both plates.

B. The neural tube gives rise to **three primary vesicles (forebrain, midbrain, and hindbrain),** which develop into **five secondary vesicles (telencephalon, diencephalon, mesencephalon, metencephalon, and myelencephalon)** (Figure 2-3).

C. **Alpha-fetoprotein (AFP)** is found in the amniotic fluid and maternal serum. It is an indicator of neural tube defects (e.g., spina bifida, anencephaly). AFP levels are reduced in mothers of fetuses with Down syndrome.

 II **The Neural Crest** (see Figure 2-1) gives rise to:

A. The **peripheral nervous system (PNS)** (i.e., peripheral nerves and sensory and autonomic ganglia).

B. The following cells:
   1. **Pseudounipolar cells of the spinal and cranial nerve** ganglia
   2. **Schwann cells** (which elaborate the myelin sheath)
   3. **Multipolar cells** of autonomic ganglia

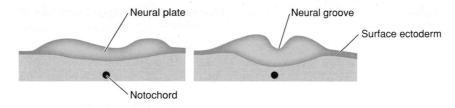

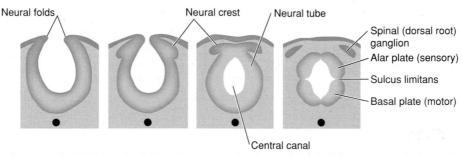

Figure 2-1 Development of the neural tube and crest.

4. Cells of the **leptomeninges** (the pia-arachnoid), which envelop the brain and spinal cord
5. **Chromaffin cells** of the suprarenal medulla (which elaborate epinephrine)
6. **Pigment cells** (melanocytes)
7. **Odontoblasts** (which elaborate predentin)
8. Cells of the **aorticopulmonary septum** of the **heart**
9. **Parafollicular cells** (calcitonin-producing C-cells)
10. **Skeletal** and **connective tissue** components of the **pharyngeal arches**

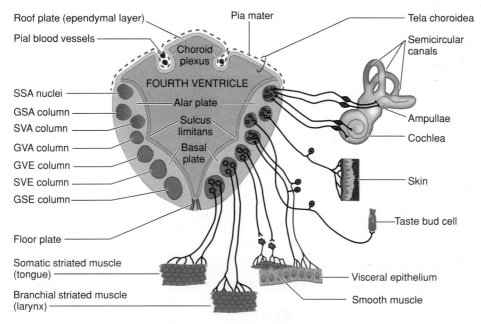

Figure 2-2 The brainstem showing the cell columns derived from the alar and basal plates. The seven cranial nerve modalities are shown. *GSA,* general somatic afferent; *GSE,* general somatic efferent; *GVA,* general visceral afferent; *GVE,* general visceral efferent; *SSA,* special somatic afferent; *SVA,* special visceral afferent; *SVE,* special visceral efferent. (Adapted from Patten BM. *Human Embryology.* 3rd ed. New York: McGraw-Hill; 1969:298, with permission.)

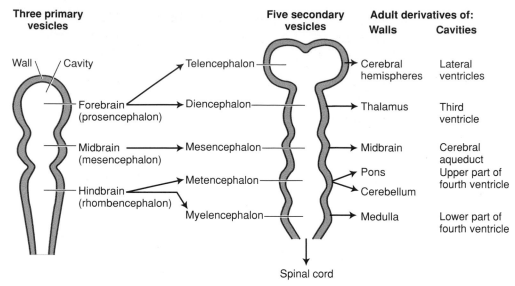

Figure 2-3 The brain vesicles indicating the adult derivatives of their walls and cavities. (Reprinted from Moore KL. *The Developing Human: Clinically Orienting Embryology.* 4th ed. Philadelphia, PA: WB Saunders; 1988:380, with permission.)

III ## The Cranial Neuropore—closure of the (cranial anterior) neuropore gives rise to the lamina terminalis. **Failure to close results in anencephaly** (i.e., failure of the brain to develop).

IV ## The Caudal Neuropore—failure to close results in spina bifida (Figure 2-4).

V ## Microglia arise from blood-born monocytes.

VI ## Myelination begins in the fourth month of gestation. Myelination of the corticospinal tracts is not completed until the end of the second postnatal year, when the tracts become functional. Myelination in the cerebral association cortex continues into the third decade of life.

A. Myelination of the CNS—accomplished by oligodendrocytes.

B. Myelination of the PNS—accomplished by Schwann cells.

VII ## The Optic Nerve and Chiasma—derived from the diencephalon. The optic nerve fibers occupy the **choroid fissure.** Failure of this fissure to close results in **coloboma iridis.**

VIII ## The Hypophysis (pituitary gland)—derived from two embryologic substrata (Figures 2-5 and 2-6).

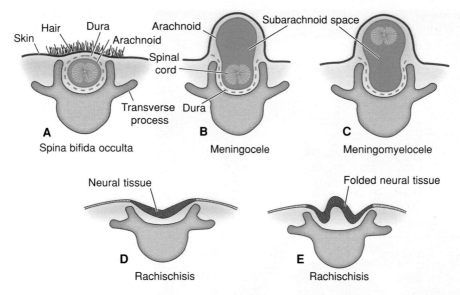

Figure 2-4 The various types of spina bifida. (Reprinted from Sadler TW. *Langman's Medical Embryology*. 6th ed. Baltimore, MD: Williams & Wilkins; 1990:363, with permission.)

A. Adenohypophysis (anterior lobe)—derived from an ectodermal diverticulum of the primitive mouth cavity (stomodeum), which is also called **Rathke pouch.** Remnants of Rathke pouch may give rise to a congenital cystic tumor, a **craniopharyngioma.**

B. Neurohypophysis (posterior lobe) develops from an anterior (ventral) evagination of the hypothalamus (neuroectoderm of the neural tube).

IX Congenital Malformations of the CNS

A. Anencephaly (Meroanencephaly)—results from failure of the cranial neuropore to close. As a result, the brain does not develop. The frequency of this condition is 1:1,000.

B. Spina Bifida results from failure of the (caudal posterior) neuropore to close. The defect usually occurs in the lumbosacral region. The frequency of spina bifida occulta is 10%.

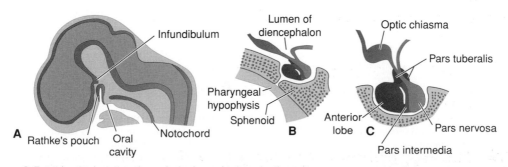

Figure 2-5 Midsagittal section through the hypophysis and sella turcica.

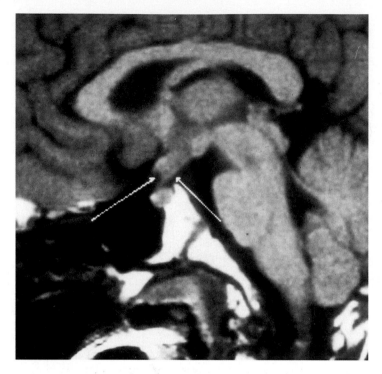

Figure 2-6 Midsagittal section through the brainstem and diencephalon. A craniopharyngioma (*arrows*) lies suprasellar in the midline. It compresses the optic chiasm and hypothalamus. This tumor is the most common supratentorial tumor that occurs in childhood and the most common cause of hypopituitarism in children. This is a T1-weighted magnetic resonance imaging scan.

C. Cranium Bifidum results from a defect in the occipital bone through which meninges, cerebellar tissue, and the fourth ventricle may herniate.

D. Chiari malformation has a frequency of 1:1,000 (Figure 2-7). It results from elongation and herniation of cerebellar tonsils through the foramen magnum, thereby blocking CSF flow.

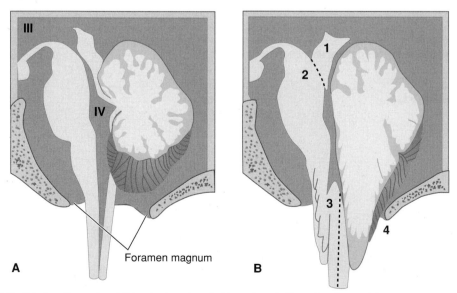

Figure 2-7 Chiari malformation. Midsagittal section. **A.** Normal cerebellum, fourth ventricle, and brainstem. **B.** Abnormal cerebellum, fourth ventricle, and brainstem showing the common congenital anomalies: (*1*) beaking of the tectal plate, (*2*) aqueductal stenosis, (*3*) kinking and transforaminal herniation of the medulla into the vertebral canal, and (*4*) herniation and unrolling of the cerebellar vermis into the vertebral canal. An accompanying meningomyelocele is common. (Reprinted from Fix JD. *BRS Neuroanatomy*. Baltimore, MD: Williams & Wilkins; 1996:72, with permission.)

E. Dandy–Walker malformation has a frequency of 1:25,000. It may result from riboflavin inhibitors, posterior fossa trauma, or viral infection (Figure 2-8).

F. Hydrocephalus—most commonly caused by stenosis of the cerebral aqueduct during development. Excessive CSF accumulates in the ventricles and subarachnoid space. This condition may result from maternal infection (cytomegalovirus and toxoplasmosis). The frequency is 1:1,000.

G. Fetal Alcohol Syndrome—the most common cause of mental retardation. It manifests with microcephaly and congenital heart disease; holoprosencephaly is the most severe manifestation.

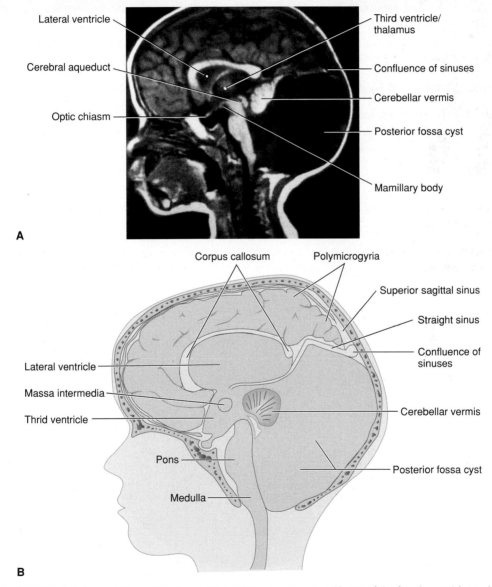

Figure 2-8 Dandy–Walker malformation. Midsagittal section. An enormous dilation of the fourth ventricle results from failure of the lateral foramina (of Luschka) and median foramen (of Magendie) to open. This condition is associated with occipital meningocele, elevation of the confluence of the sinuses (torcular Herophili), agenesis of the cerebellar vermis, and splenium of the corpus callosum. (Reprinted from Dudek RW, Fix JD. *BRS Embryology*. Baltimore, MD: Williams & Wilkins; 1997:97, with permission.)

H. Holoprosencephaly results from failure of midline cleavage of the embryonic forebrain. The telencephalon contains a singular ventricular cavity. Holoprosencephaly is seen in trisomy 13 (Patau syndrome); the corpus callosum may be absent. Holoprosencephaly is the most severe manifestation of fetal alcohol syndrome.

I. Hydranencephaly results from bilateral hemispheric infarction secondary to occlusion of the carotid arteries. The hemispheres are replaced by hugely dilated ventricles.

CASE 2-1

A mother brings her newborn infant to the clinic because the infant's "legs don't seem to work right." The infant was delivered at home without antenatal care. What is the most likely diagnosis?

Relevant Physical Exam Findings

- Tufts of hair in the lumbosacral region
- Clubfoot (Talipes equinovarus)
- Chronic upper motor neuron signs, including spasticity, weakness, and fatigability

Diagnosis

- Spina bifida occulta results from incomplete closure of the neural tube during week 4 of embryonic development. This type of neural tube defect often affects tissues overlying the spinal cord, including the vertebral column and skin.

CHAPTER 3

Neurohistology

Objectives

1. Classify neurons according to their morphology.
2. Recognize unique structural and functional characteristics of neurons.
3. List the various types of neuroglia and include a description of each along with a description of the various types of gliomas.
4. Describe the processes of nerve cell degeneration and regeneration.
5. List the types of axonal transport and the mechanisms associated with each type.
6. Describe the types of peripheral nervous system (PNS) receptors and include characteristics such as adaption level, modality, and fiber types associated with each.

 I Neurons—classified by the number of processes (Figure 3-1).

A. Pseudounipolar Neurons located in the spinal (posterior root) ganglia and sensory ganglia of cranial nerves (CNs V, VII, IX, and X).

B. Bipolar Neurons found in the cochlear and vestibular ganglia of CN VIII, in the olfactory nerve (CN I), and in the retina.

C. Multipolar Neurons the largest population of nerve cells in the nervous system. This group includes motor neurons, neurons of the autonomic nervous system, interneurons, pyramidal cells of the cerebral cortex, and Purkinje cells of the cerebellar cortex.

 II Nissl Substance—is characteristic of neurons. It consists of rosettes of polysomes and rough endoplasmic reticulum; therefore, it has a role in protein synthesis. Nissl substance is found in the **nerve cell body (perikaryon)** and **dendrites,** not in the axon hillock or axon.

 III Axonal Transport—mediates the intracellular distribution of secretory proteins, organelles, and cytoskeletal elements. It is inhibited by **colchicine,** which depolymerizes microtubules.

A. Fast Anterograde Axonal Transport—responsible for transporting all newly synthesized membranous organelles (vesicles) and precursors of neurotransmitters. This process occurs at the rate of 200 to 400 mm/day. It is mediated by neurotubules and **kinesin.** (Fast transport is neurotubule-dependent.)

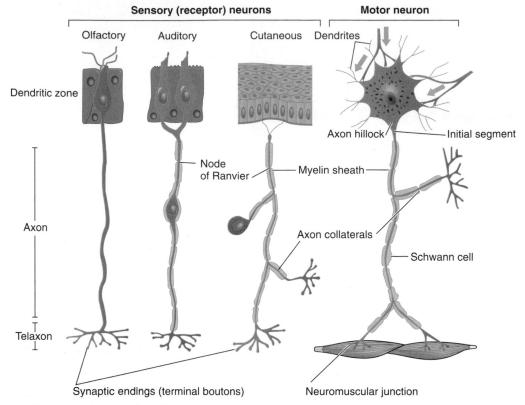

Figure 3-1 Types of nerve cells. Olfactory neurons are bipolar and unmyelinated. Auditory neurons are bipolar and myelinated. Spinal (posterior root) ganglion cells (cutaneous) are pseudounipolar and myelinated. Motor neurons are multipolar and myelinated. *Arrows* indicate input through the axons of other neurons. (Modified from Carpenter MB, Sutin J. *Human Neuroanatomy*. Baltimore, MD: Williams & Wilkins; 1983:92, with permission.)

B. Slow Anterograde Transport—responsible for transporting fibrillar cytoskeletal and proto-plasmic elements. This process occurs at the rate of 1 to 5 mm/day.

C. Fast Retrograde Transport—returns used materials from the axon terminal to the cell body for degradation and recycling at a rate of 100 to 200 mm/day. It transports **nerve growth factor, neurotropic viruses,** and toxins, such as **herpes simplex, rabies, poliovirus,** and **tetanus toxin.** It is mediated by neurotubules and **dynein.**

IV   Anterograde (Wallerian) Degeneration—characterized by the disappearance of axons and myelin sheaths and the secondary proliferation of Schwann cells. It occurs in the central nervous system (CNS) and the peripheral nervous system (PNS).

V   Chromatolysis—the result of retrograde degeneration in the neurons of the CNS and PNS. There is a loss of Nissl substance after **axotomy.**

VI   Regeneration of Nerve Cells

A. CNS. Effective regeneration does not occur in the CNS; as, there are no basement membranes or endoneural investments surrounding the axons of the CNS.

B. PNS. Regeneration is possible in the PNS. The proximal tip of a severed axon may grow into the endoneural tube, which consists of Schwann cell basement membrane and endoneurium. The axon sprout grows at the rate of 3 mm/day (Figure 3-2).

 Neuroglia—the nonneuronal cells of the nervous system.

A. Macroglia consist of astrocytes and oligodendrocytes.
   1. Astrocytes perform the following functions:
      a. Project foot processes that envelop the basement membrane of capillaries, neurons, and synapses.
      b. Form the external and internal glial-limiting membranes of the CNS.
      c. Play a role in the metabolism of certain neurotransmitters (e.g., γ-aminobutyric acid (GABA), serotonin, glutamate).
      d. Buffer the potassium concentration of the extracellular space.
      e. Form glial scars in damaged areas of the brain (i.e., astrogliosis).
      f. Contain glial fibrillary acidic protein (GFAP), which is a marker for astrocytes.
      g. Contain glutamine synthetase, another biochemical marker for astrocytes.
      h. May be identified with monoclonal antibodies (e.g., A_2B_5).
   2. Oligodendrocytes—the myelin-forming cells of the CNS. One oligodendrocyte can myelinate as many as 30 axonal segments.

B. Microglia arise from monocytes and function as the scavenger cells (phagocytes) of the CNS.

C. Ependymal Cells—ciliated cells that line the central canal and ventricles of the brain. They also line the luminal surface of the choroid plexus. **Produce cerebrospinal fluid (CSF).**

D. Tanycytes—modified ependymal cells that contact capillaries and neurons.
   ● Mediate cellular transport between the ventricles and the neuropil.
   ● Project to hypothalamic nuclei that regulate the release of gonadotropic hormone from the adenohypophysis.

E. Schwann Cells—derived from the neural crest.
   ● Myelin-forming cells of the PNS.
   ● One Schwann cell can myelinate only one internode.
   ● Schwann cells invest all myelinated and unmyelinated axons of the PNS and are separated from each other by the **nodes of Ranvier.**

 The Blood–Brain Barrier consists of the tight junctions of nonfenestrated endothelial cells and astrocytic foot processes. **Infarction of brain tissue** destroys the tight junctions of endothelial cells and results in **vasogenic edema**—an infiltrate of plasma into the extracellular space.

 The Blood–CSF Barrier consists of the tight junctions between the cuboidal epithelial cells of the choroid plexus. The barrier is permeable to some circulating peptides (e.g., insulin) and plasma proteins (e.g., prealbumin).

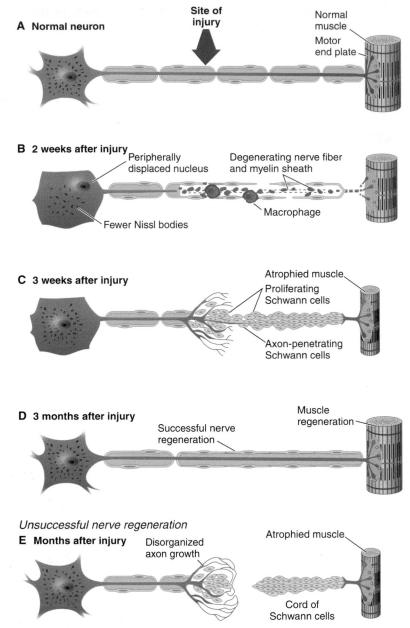

Figure 3-2 Schematic diagram of peripheral nerve regeneration.

ⓧ Pigments and Inclusions

A. Lipofuscin (Lipochrome) Granules—pigmented cytoplasmic inclusions that commonly accumulate with aging. They are considered residual bodies that are derived from lysosomes.

B. Neuromelanin (Melanin)—blackish intracytoplasmic pigment found in the substantia nigra and locus ceruleus. It disappears from nigral neurons in patients who have Parkinson disease.

C. Lewy Bodies—neuronal inclusions that are characteristic of Parkinson disease.

D. Negri Bodies—intracytoplasmic inclusions that are pathognomonic of rabies. Found in the pyramidal cells of the hippocampus and the Purkinje cells of the cerebellum.

E. Hirano Bodies—intraneuronal, eosinophilic, rodlike inclusions that are found in the hippocampus of patients with Alzheimer disease.

F. Neurofibrillary Tangles consist of intracytoplasmic degenerated neurofilaments. Seen in patients with Alzheimer disease.

G. Cowdry Type A Inclusion Bodies are intranuclear inclusions that are found in neurons and glia in herpes simplex encephalitis.

 XI **Classification of Nerve Fibers** is shown in Table 3-1.

 XII **Tumors of the CNS and PNS** are shown in Figures 3-3 and 3-4. In adults, 70% of tumors are supratentorial, while in children, 70% are infratentorial.

A. Metastatic brain tumors are more common than primary brain tumors, with the primary site of malignancy is the lung in 35% of cases, the breast in 17%, the gastrointestinal tract in 6%, melanoma in 6%, and the kidney in 5%.

B. Brain tumors are classified as glial or nonglial.

Table 3-1: Classification of Nerve Fibers

Fiber	Diameter (mm)[a]	Conduction Velocity (m/sec)	Function
Sensory Axons			
Ia (A-α)	12–20	70–120	Proprioception, muscle spindles
Ib (A-α)	12–20	70–120	Proprioception, Golgi tendon, organs
II (A-β)	5–12	30–70	Touch, pressure, and vibration
III (A-δ)	2–5	12–30	Touch, pressure, fast pain, and temperature
IV (C)	0.5–1	0.5–2	Slow pain and temperature, unmyelinated fibers
Motor Axons			
Alpha (A-α)	12–20	15–120	Alpha motor neurons of anterior horn (innervate extrafusal muscle fibers)
Gamma (A-γ)	2–10	10–45	Gamma motor neurons of anterior horn (innervate intrafusal muscle fibers)
Preganglionic autonomic fibers (B)	<3	3–15	Myelinated preganglionic autonomic fibers
Postganglionic autonomic fibers (C)	1	2	Unmyelinated postganglionic autonomic fibers

[a]Myelin sheath included if present.

Germinomas
- germ cell tumors commonly seen in pineal region (> 50%)
- overlie tectum of midbrain
- cause obstructive hydrocephalus due to aqueductal stenosis
- common cause of Parinaud's syndrome

Meningiomas
- derived from arachnoid cap cells and represent second most common primary intracranial brain tumor after astrocytomas (15%)
- are not invasive; they indent brain; may produce hyperostosis
- pathology: concentric whorls and calcified psammoma bodies
- location: parasagittal and convexity
- gender: females > males
- associated with neurofibromatosis-2 (NF-2)

Brain abscesses
- may result from sinusitis, mastoiditis, hematogenous spread
- location: frontal and temporal lobes, cerebellum
- organisms; streptococci, staphylococci, and pneumococci
- result in cerebral edema and herniation

Astrocytomas
- represent 20% of gliomas
- histologically benign
- diffusely infiltrate hemispheric white matter
- most common glioma found in posterior fossa of children

Ependymomas

Glioblastoma multiforme
- represents 55% of gliomas
- malignant; rapidly fatal astrocytic tumor
- commonly found in frontal and temporal lobes and basal nuclei
- frequently crosses midline via corpus callosum (butterfly glioma)
- most common primary brain tumor
- histology: pseudopalisades, perivascular pseudorosettes

Colloid cysts of third ventricle
- comprise 2% of intracranial gliomas
- are of ependymal origin
- found at interventricular foramina
- ventricular obstruction results in increased intracranial pressure and may cause positional headaches, "drop attacks," or sudden death

Oligodendrogliomas
- represent 5% of all gliomas
- grows slowly and are relatively benign
- most common in frontal lobe
- calcification in 50% of cases
- cells look like fried eggs (perinuclear halos)

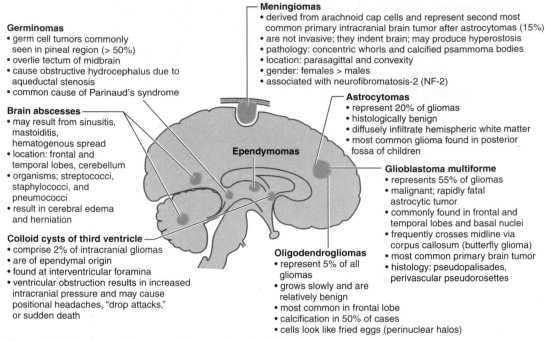

Figure 3-3 Supratentorial tumors of the central and peripheral nervous systems.

Choroid plexus papillomas
- histology: benign; no necrosis or invasive features
- represent 2% of the gliomas
- one of the most common brain tumors in patients <2 years of age
- occur in decreasing frequency: fourth, lateral, and third ventricle
- CSF overproduction may cause hydrocephalus

Craniopharyngiomas
- represent 3% of primary brain tumors
- derived from epithelial remnants of Rathke pouch
- location: suprasellar and inferior to optic chiasma
- cause bitemporal hemianopia and hypopituitarism
- calcification is common

Cerebellar astrocytomas
- benign tumors of childhood with good prognosis
- most common pediatric intracranial tumor
- contain pilocytic astrocytes and Rosenthal fibers

Pituitary adenomas (PA)
- most common tumors of pituitary gland
- prolactinoma is most common PA
- derived from the stomodeum (Rathke pouch)
- represent 8% of primary brain tumors
- may cause hypopituitarism, visual field defects (bitemporal hemianopia and cranial nerve palsies CN III, IV, VI, V$_1$ and V$_2$, and postganglionic sympathetic fibers to dilator pupillae

Medulloblastomas
- represent 7% of primary brain tumors
- represent primitive neuroectodermal tumors (PNET)
- second most common posterior fossa tumor in children
- responsible for posterior vermis syndrome
- can metastasize via CSF tracts
- highly radiosensitive

Hemangioblastomas
- characterized by abundant capillary blood vessels and foamy cells; most often found in cerebellum
- when found in cerebellum and retina, may represent part of von Hippel-Lindau syndrome
- 2% of primary intracranial tumors; 10% of posterior fossa tumors

Schwannomas (acoustic neuromas)
- consist of Schwann cells and arise from vestibular division of CN VIII
- comprise approx. 8% of intracranial neoplasms
- pathology: Antoni A and B tissue and Verocay bodies
- bilateral acoustic neuromas are diagnostic of NF-2
- gender: females > males

Brainstem glioma
- usually benign pilocytic astrocytoma
- usually causes cranial nerve palsies
- may cause "locked-in" syndrome

Intraspinal tumors
- Schwannomas 30%
- Meningiomas 25%
- Gliomas 20%
- Sarcomas 12%
- Ependymomas represent 60% of intramedullary gliomas

Ependymomas
- represent 5% of the gliomas
- histology: benign, ependymal tubules, perivascular pseudorosettes
- 40% are supratentorial; 60% are infratentorial (posterior fossa)
- most common spinal cord glioma (60%)
- third most common posterior fossa tumor in children and adolescents

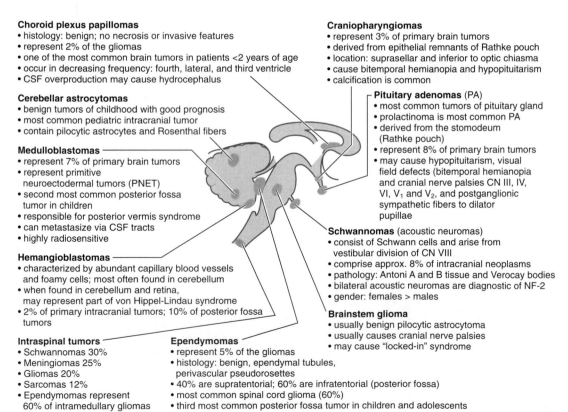

Figure 3-4 Infratentorial (posterior fossa) and intraspinal tumors of the central and peripheral nervous systems.

C. The five most common brain tumors are:
1. **Glioblastoma multiforme,** the most common and most fatal type.
2. **Meningioma,** a benign noninvasive tumor of the falx and the convexity of the hemisphere.
3. **Schwannoma,** a benign peripheral tumor derived from Schwann cells.
4. **Ependymoma,** found in the ventricles and accounts for 60% of spinal cord gliomas.
5. **Medulloblastoma,** the second most common posterior fossa tumor seen in children and may metastasize through the CSF tracts.

 XIII **Cutaneous Receptors** **(Figure 3-5)**—divided into two large groups: free nerve endings and encapsulated endings.

A. Free nerve endings are nociceptors (pain) and thermoreceptors (cold and heat).

B. Encapsulated endings are touch receptors (Meissner corpuscles) and pressure and vibration receptors (Pacinian corpuscles).

C. Merkel disks are unencapsulated light touch receptors.

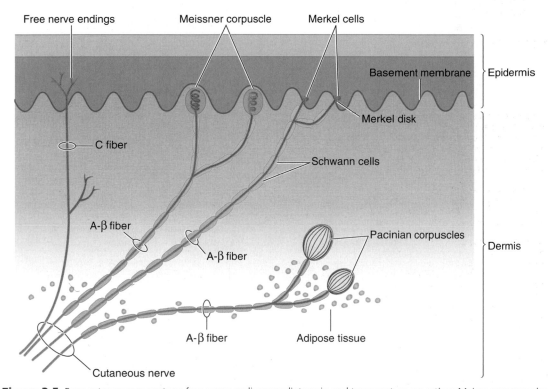

Figure 3-5 Four cutaneous receptors: free nerve endings mediate pain and temperature sensation; Meissner corpuscles of the dermal papillae mediate tactile two-point discrimination; Pacinian corpuscles of the dermis mediate touch, pressure, and vibration sensation; Merkel disks mediate light touch.

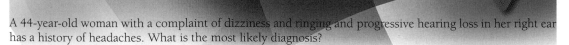

CASE 3-1

A 44-year-old woman with a complaint of dizziness and ringing and progressive hearing loss in her right ear has a history of headaches. What is the most likely diagnosis?

Relevant Physical Exam Findings

- Unilateral sensorineural hearing loss

Relevant Lab Findings

- Radiologic findings show a right cerebellopontine angle mass that involves the pons and cerebellum.
- Neurologic workup shows discrimination impairment out of proportion to pure-tone thresholds.

Diagnosis

- Acoustic schwannomas are intracranial tumors that arise from the Schwann cells investing CN VIII (the vestibulocochlear nerve). They account for up to 90% of tumors found within the cerebellopontine angle. Cranial nerves V and VII are the next most common nerves of origin of schwannomas.

CHAPTER 4

Blood Supply

Objectives

1. List the major branches of the vertebral and internal carotid arteries and indicate the regions/structures that each artery supplies.
2. Describe the cerebral arterial circle (of Willis).
3. List the major deep cerebral veins.
4. Explain and identify the dural venous sinuses and include a description of their drainage patterns and location of each sinus.
5. Describe the various types of intracranial hemorrhage.

 I **The Spinal Cord and Caudal Brainstem** are supplied with blood through the anterior spinal artery (Figure 4-1).

A. The anterior spinal artery supplies the **anterior two-thirds of the spinal cord.**

B. In the **medulla,** the anterior spinal artery supplies the pyramid, medial lemniscus, and root fibers of cranial nerve (CN XII).

 II **The Internal Carotid System** (see Figure 4-1) consists of the **internal carotid artery** and its branches:

A. Ophthalmic Artery enters the orbit with the optic nerve (CN II). The **central artery of the retina** is a branch of the ophthalmic artery. Occlusion results in blindness.

B. Posterior Communicating Artery irrigates the hypothalamus and ventral thalamus. An **aneurysm** of this artery is the second most common aneurysm of the cerebral arterial circle and commonly results in **third-nerve palsy.**

C. Anterior Choroidal Artery arises from the internal carotid artery. It perfuses the lateral geniculate body, globus pallidus, and posterior limb of the internal capsule.

D. Anterior Cerebral Artery (Figure 4-2) supplies the medial surface of the cerebral hemisphere from the frontal pole to the parieto-occipital sulcus.
   1. The anterior cerebral artery irrigates the **paracentral lobule,** which contains the leg-foot area of the motor and sensory cortices.
   2. The **anterior communicating artery** connects the two anterior cerebral arteries. It is the most common site of **aneurysm** of the cerebral arterial circle, which may cause **bitemporal lower quadrantanopia.**

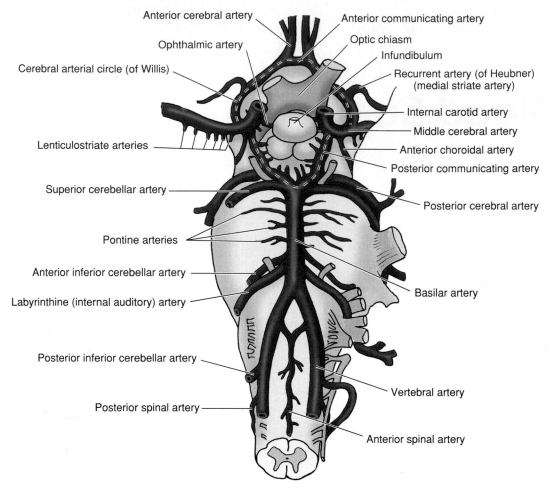

Figure 4-1 Arterial supply to the brain as seen from the undersurface of the brainstem.

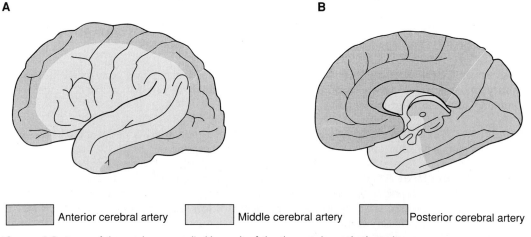

Figure 4-2 Areas of the cerebrum supplied by each of the three main cerebral arteries.

Medial

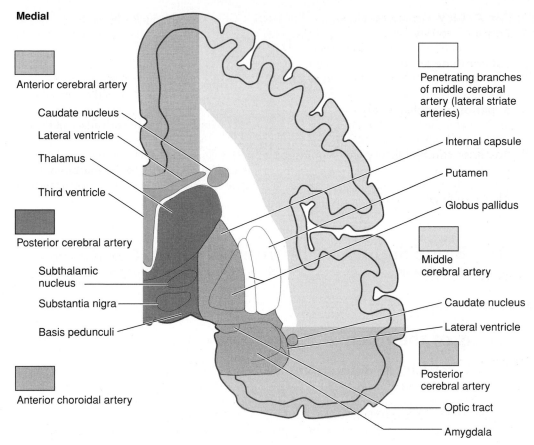

Anterior cerebral artery

Caudate nucleus

Lateral ventricle

Thalamus

Third ventricle

Posterior cerebral artery

Subthalamic nucleus

Substantia nigra

Basis pedunculi

Anterior choroidal artery

Penetrating branches of middle cerebral artery (lateral striate arteries)

Internal capsule

Putamen

Globus pallidus

Middle cerebral artery

Caudate nucleus

Lateral ventricle

Posterior cerebral artery

Optic tract

Amygdala

Figure 4-3 Coronal section through the cerebral hemisphere at the level of the internal capsule and thalamus, showing the major vascular territories.

3. The **medial striate arteries** (see Figure 4-1) are the penetrating arteries of the anterior cerebral artery. They supply the anterior portion of the putamen and caudate nucleus and the anteroinferior part of the internal capsule.

E. Middle Cerebral Artery (Figure 4-2)

1. Supplies the lateral convexity of the hemisphere, including:
  a. Broca and Wernicke speech areas.
  b. The **face** and **arm areas** of the motor and sensory cortices.
  c. The **frontal eye field.**
2. Lateral striate arteries (Figure 4-3)—penetrating branches of the middle cerebral artery. They are the arteries of **stroke,** and they supply the **internal capsule, caudate nucleus, putamen, and globus pallidus.**

III The Vertebrobasilar System. See Figure 4-1.

A. Vertebral Artery—a branch of the subclavian artery. Gives rise to the **anterior spinal artery** (see section I) and the **posterior inferior cerebellar artery (PICA),** which supplies the dorsolateral quadrant of the medulla. This quadrant includes the nucleus ambiguus (CNs IX and X) and the inferior surface of the cerebellum.

B. Basilar Artery—formed by the two vertebral arteries. Gives rise to the following arteries:

1. **Pontine arteries** supply the base of the pons, which includes the corticospinal fibers and the exiting root fibers of the abducent nerve (CN VI).
2. **Labyrinthine artery** supplies structures of the inner ear.
3. **Anterior inferior cerebellar artery (AICA)** supplies the caudal lateral pontine tegmentum, including CN VII, the spinal trigeminal tract of CN V, and the inferior surface of the cerebellum.
4. **Superior cerebellar artery** supplies the dorsolateral tegmentum of the rostral pons (i.e., rostral to the motor nucleus of CN V), the superior cerebellar peduncle, the superior surface of the cerebellum and cerebellar nuclei, and the cochlear nuclei.
5. **Posterior cerebral artery (see Figures 4-1 to 4-3)** is connected to the carotid artery through the posterior communicating artery. It provides the **major blood supply to the midbrain.** It also supplies the thalamus and the occipital lobe. **Occlusion** of this artery results in a **contralateral hemianopia with macular sparing.**

IV The Blood Supply of the Internal Capsule comes primarily from the **lateral striate arteries** of the middle cerebral artery and the **anterior choroidal artery.**

V Veins of the Brain (see Figures 4-4 and 4-13)

A. Superior Cerebral ("Bridging") Veins drain into the superior sagittal sinus. Laceration results in a **subdural hematoma (SDH).** Sudden deceleration of the head causes tearing of the superior cerebral veins. SDH extends over the crest of the convexity of the brain into the interhemispheric fissure but does not cross the dural attachment of the falx cerebri. The clot can be crescent-shaped, biconvex, or multiloculated. SDHs are more common than epidural hematomas and always cause brain damage.

B. Great Cerebral Vein (of Galen) drains the deep cerebral veins into the **straight sinus.**

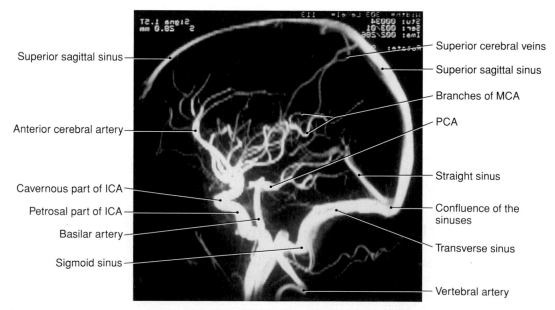

Figure 4-4 Magnetic resonance angiogram, lateral projection, showing the major venous sinuses and arteries. Note the bridging veins entering the superior sagittal sinus. *ICA,* internal carotid artery; *MCA,* middle cerebral artery; *PCA,* posterior cerebral artery.

VI Venous Dural Sinuses

A. Superior Sagittal Sinus receives blood from the bridging veins and **emissary veins** (a potential route for transmission of extracranial infection into the brain). The superior sagittal sinus also receives cerebrospinal fluid (CSF) through the arachnoid villi.

B. Cavernous Sinus contains CNs III, IV, V_1 and V_2, and VI and the postganglionic sympathetic fibers. It also contains the siphon of the internal carotid artery (Figure 4-4).

VII Angiography

A. Carotid Angiography. Figure 4-5A,B shows the internal carotid artery, anterior cerebral artery, and middle cerebral artery.

B. Vertebral Angiography. Figure 4-5C,D shows the vertebral artery, PICA and AICA, basilar artery, superior cerebellar artery, and posterior cerebral artery (Figures 4-6 and 4-7).

C. Veins and Dural Sinuses. Figure 4-7 shows the internal cerebral vein, superior cerebral veins, great cerebral vein, superior ophthalmic vein, and major dural sinuses.

D. Digital Subtraction Angiography. See Figures 4-8 to 4-11.

VIII The Middle Meningeal Artery, a branch of the maxillary artery,

enters the cranium through the **foramen spinosum.** It supplies most of the dura, including its calvarial portion. Laceration results in **epidural hemorrhage** (hematoma) (Figures 4-12 and 4-13). A classic "lucid interval" is seen in 50% of cases.

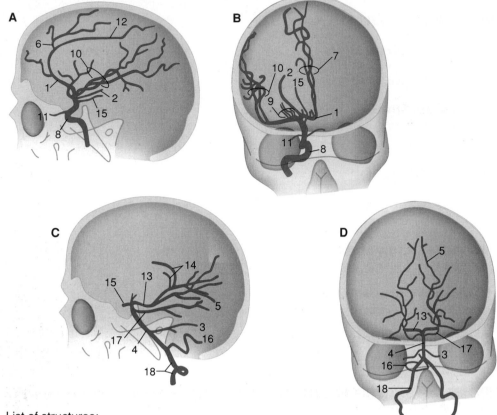

List of structures:

1. Anterior cerebral artery
2. Anterior choroidal artery
3. Anterior inferior cerebellar artery
4. Basilar artery
5. Calcarine artery
6 Callosomarginal artery
7. Callosmarginal and pericallosal arteries
   (of anterior cerebral artery)
8. Internal carotid artery
9. Lateral striate arteries

10. Middle cerebral artery
11. Ophthalmic artery
12. Pericallosal artery
13. Posterior cerebral artery
14. Posterior choridal arteries
15. Posterior communicating artery
16. Posterior inferior cerebellar artery
17. Superior cerebellar artery
18. Vertebral artery

Figure 4-5 **A.** Carotid angiogram, lateral projection. **B.** Carotid angiogram, anteroposterior projection. **C.** Vertebral angiogram, lateral projection. **D.** Vertebral angiogram, anteroposterior projection.

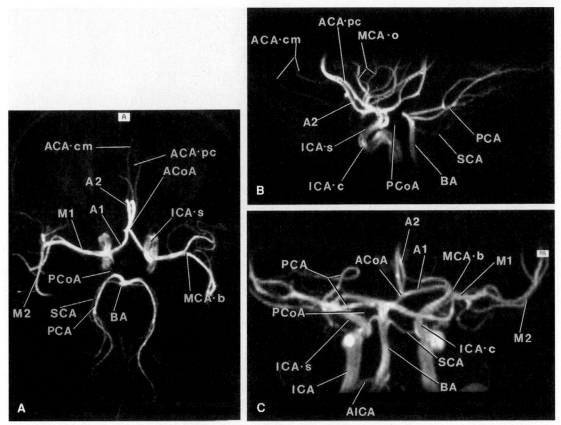

Figure 4-6 Arterial anatomy of a magnetic resonance section; axial **(A),** sagittal **(B, C).** *ACAcm,* anterior cerebral artery, callosal marginal branch; *A2* and *A1,* branches of the anterior cerebral artery; *ACApc,* pericallosal branch of the anterior cerebral artery; *ACoA,* anterior communicating artery; *AICA,* anterior inferior cerebellar artery; *M1* and *M2,* segments of the middle cerebral artery *(MCA);* *MCAb,* bifurcation; *ICAs,* internal carotid artery siphon; *ICAc,* internal carotid artery cavernous; *PCA,* posterior cerebral artery; *PCoA,* posterior communicating artery; *BA,* basilar artery; *SCA,* superior cerebellar artery. (Reprinted from Grossman CB, *Magnetic Resonance Imaging and Computed Tomography of the Head and Spine.* 2nd ed. Philadelphia, PA: Williams & Wilkins; 1996:124, with permission.)

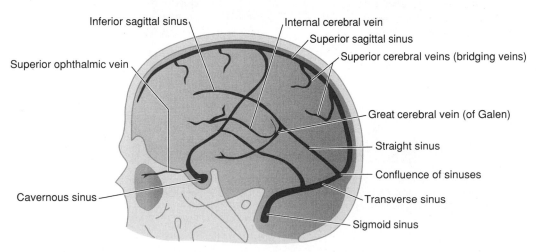

Figure 4-7 Carotid angiogram, venous phase, showing the cerebral veins and venous sinuses.

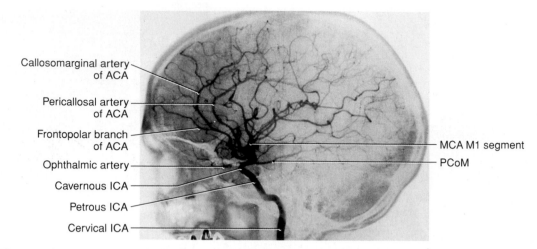

Callosomarginal artery of ACA

Pericallosal artery of ACA

Frontopolar branch of ACA

Ophthalmic artery

Cavernous ICA

Petrous ICA

Cervical ICA

MCA M1 segment

PCoM

Figure 4-8 Carotid angiogram, lateral projection. Identify the cortical branches of the anterior cerebral artery (*ACA*) and middle cerebral artery (*MCA*). Follow the course of the internal carotid artery (*ICA*). Remember that aneurysms of the posterior communicating artery (*PCoM*) may result in third-nerve palsy. The paracentral lobule is irrigated by the callosomarginal artery.

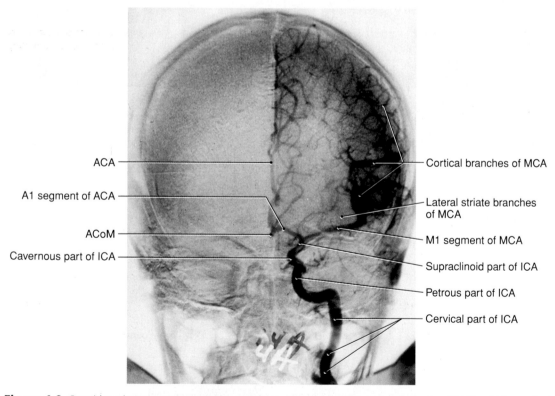

ACA

A1 segment of ACA

ACoM

Cavernous part of ICA

Cortical branches of MCA

Lateral striate branches of MCA

M1 segment of MCA

Supraclinoid part of ICA

Petrous part of ICA

Cervical part of ICA

Figure 4-9 Carotid angiogram, anteroposterior projection. Identify the anterior cerebral artery (*ACA*), middle cerebral artery (*MCA*), and internal carotid artery (*ICA*). The horizontal branches of the MCA perfuse the basal nuclei and internal capsule. *ACoM,* anterior communicating artery.

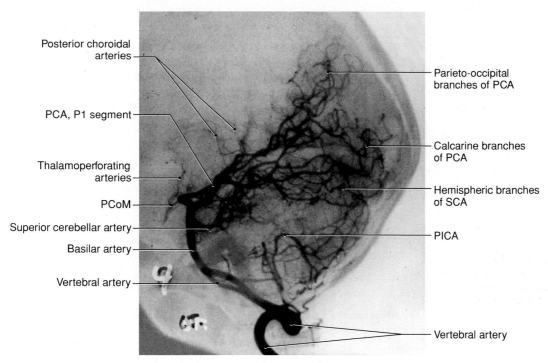

Posterior choroidal arteries

PCA, P1 segment

Thalamoperforating arteries

PCoM

Superior cerebellar artery

Basilar artery

Vertebral artery

Parieto-occipital branches of PCA

Calcarine branches of PCA

Hemispheric branches of SCA

PICA

Vertebral artery

Figure 4-10 Vertebral angiogram, lateral projection. Two structures are found between the posterior cerebral artery (*PCA*) and the superior cerebellar artery (*SCA*): the tentorium and the third cranial nerve. *PCoM,* posterior communicating artery; *PICA,* posterior inferior cerebellar artery.

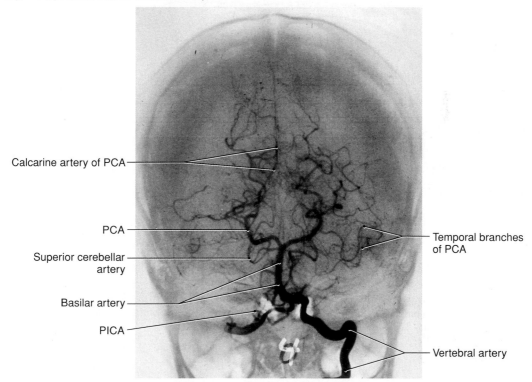

Calcarine artery of PCA

PCA

Superior cerebellar artery

Basilar artery

PICA

Temporal branches of PCA

Vertebral artery

Figure 4-11 Vertebral angiogram, anteroposterior projection. Which artery supplies the visual cortex? The calcarine artery, a branch of the posterior cerebral artery (*PCA*). Occlusion of the PCA (calcarine artery) results in a contralateral homonymous hemianopia, with macular sparing. *PICA,* posterior inferior cerebellar artery.

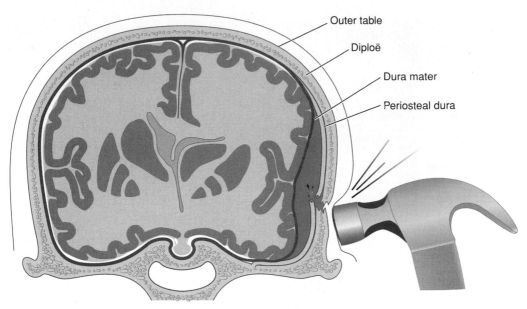

Figure 4-12 An epidural hematoma results from laceration of the middle meningeal artery. Note the biconvex clot. (Reprinted from Osburn AG, Tong KA. *Handbook of Neuroradiology: Brain and Skull*. St. Louis, MO: Mosby; 1996:191, with permission.)

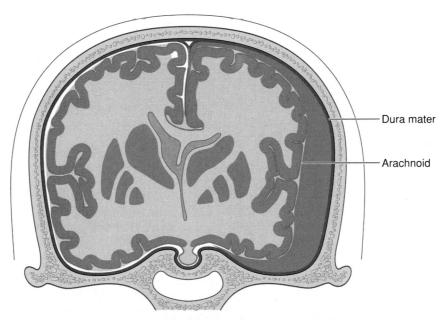

Figure 4-13 A subdural hematoma (SDH) results from lacerated bridging veins. SDHs are frequently accompanied by traumatic subarachnoid hemorrhages and cortical contusions. (Reprinted from Osburn AG, Tong KA. *Handbook of Neuroradiology: Brain and Skull*. St. Louis, MO: Mosby; 1996:192, with permission.)

CASE 4-1

A 62-year-old man comes to the clinic complaining of problems with his vision and a horrible headache that began earlier in the day. He reports bumping into objects and not being able to read half the printed page of the newspaper. He has a history of hypertension and diabetes mellitus. What is the most likely diagnosis?

Relevant Physical Exam Findings

- Complete hemianopia
- Contralateral face and limb sensory loss

Relevant Lab Findings

- Computed tomography scan of the brain determined the presence of ischemic infarction with hemorrhagic change.

Diagnosis

- Posterior cerebral artery infarct

CHAPTER 5

Meninges, Ventricles, and Cerebrospinal Fluid

Objectives

1. Describe the location and identifying characteristics of the dura mater, arachnoid, and pia mater.
2. Explain where cerebrospinal fluid (CSF) is created and the route it takes to the systemic circulation.
3. Identify the ventricles and list the subdivisions and characteristics of each.
4. Describe the flow of CSF through the ventricular system.
5. Identify the meningeal spaces and include a description of what is found in each, and whether the spaces are real or potential.
6. Describe the various types of hydrocephalus and meningitis, along with their causes and findings.

 Meninges—three **connective tissue membranes** that surround the spinal cord and brain.

A. Consist of the **pia mater, arachnoid mater,** and **dura mater.**

1. **Pia mater**—delicate, highly vascular layer of connective tissue. Closely covers the surface of the brain and spinal cord.
2. **Arachnoid mater**—delicate, avascular connective tissue membrane. Located between the dura mater and the pia mater. Loosely adhered to the dura mater by **dural border cells** and the pressure of the underlying cerebrospinal fluid (CSF).
3. **Dura mater**—outer layer of meninges. Consists of dense connective tissue that is divided into an outer periosteal (endosteal) layer and an inner meningeal layer. In the cranial vault, the meningeal layer forms dural folds and forms the dura mater of the spinal cord. Dural venous sinuses are located between periosteal and meningeal layers of dura mater.

B. Meningeal Spaces

1. **Subarachnoid space (Figure 5-1)** lies between the pia mater and the arachnoid.
   a. Terminates at the level of the second sacral vertebra.
   b. Contains the CSF.
2. **Subdural space**
   a. In the **cranium,** the subdural space is traversed by "bridging" veins.
   b. In the **spinal cord,** it is a clinically insignificant potential space.
3. **Epidural space**
   a. **Cranial epidural space** is a potential space. It contains the meningeal arteries and veins.
   b. **Spinal epidural space** contains fatty areolar tissue, lymphatics, and venous plexuses. The epidural space may be injected with a local anesthetic to produce a paravertebral ("saddle") nerve block.

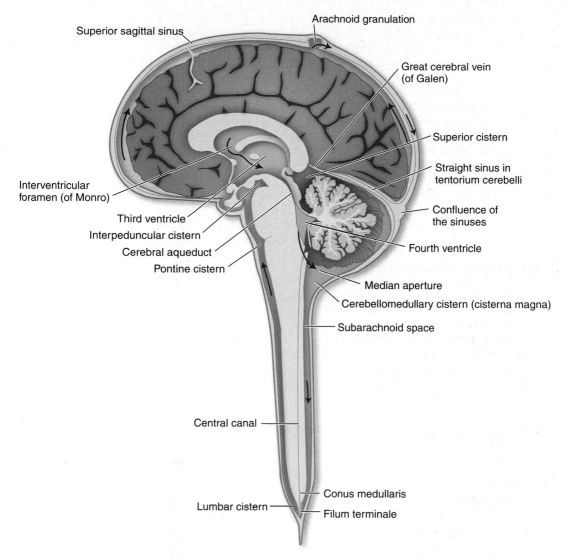

Figure 5-1 The subarachnoid spaces and cisterns of the brain and spinal cord. Note that the conus medullaris terminates at L-1. The lumbar cistern ends at S-2. (Reprinted from Noback CR, Strominger NL, Demarest R. *The Human Nervous System*. 4th ed. Baltimore, MD: Williams & Wilkins; 1991:68, with permission.)

C. Meningeal Tumors

1. **Meningiomas**—benign, well-circumscribed, slow-growing tumors. They account for 15% of primary intracranial tumors and are more common in women than in men (3:2). Ninety percent of meningiomas are supratentorial.
2. **Subdural and epidural hematomas**
   a. **Subdural hematoma**—caused by laceration of the superior cerebral (bridging) veins.
   b. **Epidural hematoma**—caused by laceration of a cerebral artery, most commonly the middle meningeal artery.

D. Meningitis—inflammation of the pia-arachnoid area of the brain, the spinal cord, or both.

1. **Bacterial meningitis**—characterized clinically by fever, headache, nuchal rigidity, and Kernig sign. (With the patient supine, the examiner flexes the patient's hip but cannot extend the knee without causing pain. **(Remember: Kernig = knee.)** More than 70% of cases occur in children younger than 5 years. The disease may cause cranial nerve palsies and hydrocephalus.

a. **Common causes**
   i. *Newborns* (younger than 1 month), bacterial meningitis is most frequently caused by *group B streptococci* (*Streptococcus agalactiae*), *Escherichia coli,* and *Listeria monocytogenes.*
   ii. *Older infants and young children* (1 to 23 months)—most commonly caused by *Streptococcus pneumoniae.*
   iii. *Young adults* (2 to 18 years)—most frequently caused by *Neisseria meningitidis.*
   iv. *Older adults* (19 years and older)—most frequently caused by *S. pneumoniae.*
      Immunization against *Haemophilus influenzae* has significantly reduced this type of meningitis.
b. **CSF findings**
   i. *Numerous polymorphonuclear leukocytes*
   ii. *Decreased glucose levels*
   iii. *Increased protein levels*
2. **Viral Meningitis**—also known as aseptic meningitis. Is characterized clinically by fever, headache, nuchal rigidity, and Kernig sign.
   a. **Common causes**—many viruses are associated with viral meningitis, including mumps, echovirus, Coxsackievirus, Epstein–Barr virus, and herpes simplex type 2.
   b. **CSF findings**
      i. *Numerous lymphocytes*
      ii. *Normal glucose levels*
      iii. *Moderately increased protein levels*

II Ventricular System

A. Choroid Plexus—a specialized structure that projects into all four ventricles of the brain. Consists of infoldings of blood vessels of the pia mater that are covered by modified ciliated ependymal cells. It secretes CSF.

B. Ventricles Contain CSF and Choroid Plexus

1. Two **lateral ventricles** communicate with the third ventricle through the **interventricular foramina** (of Monro).
2. **Third ventricle**—located between the medial walls of the diencephalon. Communicates with the fourth ventricle through the cerebral aqueduct.
3. **Cerebral aqueduct** (of Sylvius) connects the third and fourth ventricles. Blockage of the cerebral aqueduct results in noncommunicating hydrocephalus.
4. **Fourth ventricle** communicates with the subarachnoid space through three outlet foramina: two **lateral foramina** (of Luschka) and one **median foramen** (of Magendie).

C. Hydrocephalus—dilation of the cerebral ventricles caused by blockage of the CSF pathways.
Characterized by excessive accumulation of CSF in the ventricles or subarachnoid space.

1. **Noncommunicating hydrocephalus** results from obstruction within the ventricles (e.g., congenital aqueductal stenosis).
2. **Communicating hydrocephalus** results from blockage within the subarachnoid space (e.g., adhesions after meningitis).
3. **Normal-pressure hydrocephalus** occurs when the CSF is not absorbed by the arachnoid villi. May occur secondary to posttraumatic meningeal hemorrhage. Characterized by the triad of progressive dementia, ataxic gait, and urinary incontinence. **(Remember: wacky, wobbly, and wet.)**
4. **Hydrocephalus ex vacuo** results from a loss of cells in the caudate nucleus (e.g., Huntington disease).
5. **Pseudotumor cerebri** (benign intracranial hypertension) results from increased resistance to CSF outflow at the arachnoid villi. Occurs in obese young women and is characterized by papilledema without mass, elevated CSF pressure, and deteriorating vision. The ventricles may be slit-like.

Table 5-1: Cerebrospinal Fluid Profiles in Subarachnoid Hemorrhage, Bacterial Meningitis, and Viral Encephalitis

Cerebrospinal Fluid	Normal	Subarachnoid Hemorrhage	Bacterial Meningitis	Viral Encephalitis
Color	Clear	Bloody	Cloudy	Clear, cloudy
Cell count/mm³	<5 lymphocytes	Red blood cells present	>1,000 polymorpho-nuclear leukocytes	25–500 lymphocytes
Protein	<45 mg/dL	Normal to slightly elevated	Elevated, >100 mg/dL	Slightly elevated
Glucose ~66% of blood (80–120 mg/dL)	>45 mg/dL	Normal	Reduced	Normal

 III ## Cerebrospinal Fluid—a colorless acellular fluid. Flows through the ventricles and into the subarachnoid space.

A. Function
1. **CSF supports the central nervous system (CNS) and protects it** against concussive injury.
2. **Transports hormones** and hormone-releasing factors.
3. **Removes metabolic waste products** through absorption.

B. Formation and Absorption—CSF is formed by the choroid plexus. Absorption is primarily through the arachnoid villi into the superior sagittal sinus.

C. Composition of CSF is clinically relevant (Table 5-1).
1. The normal number of **mononuclear cells** is fewer than 5/μL.
2. **Red blood cells** in the CSF indicate subarachnoid hemorrhage (e.g., caused by trauma or a ruptured berry aneurysm).
3. **CSF glucose** levels are normally 50 to 75 mg/dL (66% of the blood glucose level). Glucose levels are normal in patients with viral meningitis and decreased in patients with bacterial meningitis.
4. **Total protein levels** are normally between 15 and 45 mg/dL in the lumbar cistern. Protein levels are increased in patients with bacterial meningitis and normal or slightly increased in patients with viral meningitis.
5. **Normal CSF pressure** in the lateral recumbent position ranges from 80 to 180 mm H_2O.

 IV ## Herniation (Figures 5-2 to 5-7)

A. Transtentorial (Uncal) Herniation is protrusion of part of the brain through the tentorial incisure. May result in oculomotor paresis and contralateral hemiplegia.

B. Transforaminal (Tonsillar) Herniation—protrusion of the brainstem and cerebellum through the foramen magnum. Clinical complications include obtundation and death.

C. Subfalcine (Cingulate) Herniation—herniation below the falx cerebri (cerebral falx). Does not necessarily result in severe clinical symptoms. Can present as headache. Compression of the anterior cerebral artery may result in contralateral lower limb weakness.

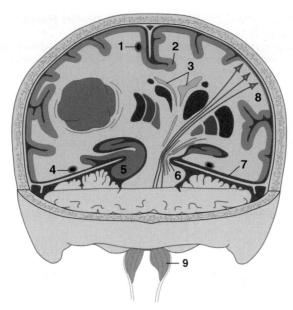

Figure 5-2 Coronal section of a tumor in the supratentorial compartment. *(1)* Anterior cerebral artery; *(2)* subfalcine herniation; *(3)* shifting of the lateral ventricles; *(4)* posterior cerebral artery (compression results in contralateral hemianopia); *(5)* uncal (transtentorial) herniation; *(6)* Kernohan notch (contralateral cerebral peduncle), with damaged corticospinal and corticonuclear fibers; *(7)* tentorium cerebelli; *(8)* pyramidal cells that give rise to the corticospinal tract; *(9)* tonsillar (transforaminal) herniation, which damages vital medullary centers. (Adapted with permission from Leech RW, Shumann RM. *Neuropathology*. New York: Harper & Row; 1982:16.)

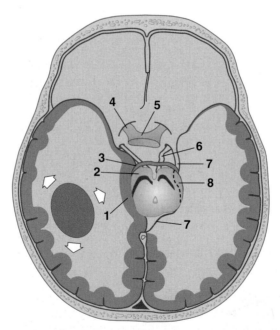

Figure 5-3 Axial section through the midbrain and the herniating parahippocampal gyrus. The left oculomotor nerve is being stretched (dilated pupil). The left posterior cerebral artery is compressed, resulting in a contralateral hemianopia. The right crus cerebri is damaged (Kernohan notch) by the free edge of the tentorial incisure, resulting in a contralateral hemiparesis. Kernohan notch results in a false localizing sign. The caudal displacement of the brainstem causes rupture of the paramedian arteries of the basilar artery. The posterior cerebral arteries lie superior to the oculomotor nerves. (1) Parahippocampal gyrus; (2) crus cerebri; (3) posterior cerebral artery; (4) optic nerve; (5) optic chiasma; (6) oculomotor nerve; (7) free edge of tentorium; (8) Kernohan notch. (Adapted from Leech RW, Shumann RM. *Neuropathology*. New York: Harper & Row; 1982:19, with permission.)

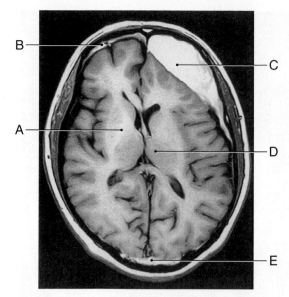

Figure 5-4 Magnetic resonance imaging scan showing brain trauma. *(A)* Internal capsule; *(B)* subdural hematoma; *(C)* subdural hematoma; *(D)* thalamus; *(E)* epidural hematoma. The hyperintense signals are caused by methemoglobin. This is a T1-weighted image.

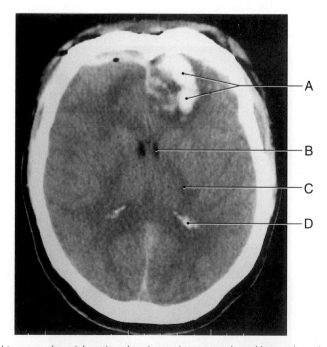

Figure 5-5 Computed tomography axial section showing an intraparenchymal hemorrhage in the left frontal lobe. *(A)* Intraparenchymal hemorrhage; *(B)* lateral ventricle; *(C)* internal capsule; *(D)* calcified glomus in the trigone region of the lateral ventricle.

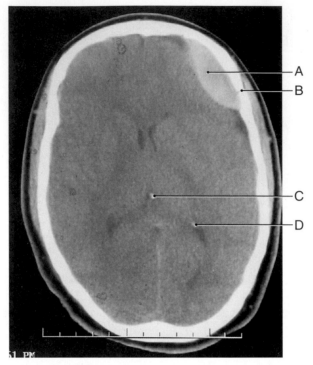

Figure 5-6 Computed tomography axial section showing an epidural hematoma and a skull fracture. *(A)* Epidural hematoma; *(B)* skull fracture; *(C)* calcified pineal gland; *(D)* calcified glomus in the trigone region of the lateral ventricle. The epidural hematoma is a classic biconvex, or lentiform, shape.

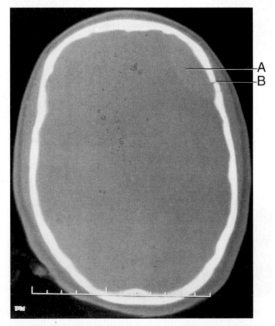

Figure 5-7 Computed tomography (CT) axial section showing a skull fracture *(A)* on the left side. An epidural hematoma *(B)* underlies the fracture. The CT scan shows a bone window.

CASE 5-1

The patient is a 68-year-old man with alcoholic cirrhosis. He fell 4 weeks ago. He has a history of progressive weakness on the right side. What is the most likely diagnosis?

Relevant Physical Exam Findings

- Hemiparesis
- Reflex asymmetry

Relevant Lab Findings

- Computed tomography scan of the head showed a crescent-shaped hypodense area between the cortex and skull. This mass has resulted in massive midline shift to the right, with subfalcine and uncal herniation.

Diagnosis

- Subdural hematoma results from bleeding between the dura mater and the arachnoid membrane from the bridging veins that connect the cerebral cortex to the dural venous sinuses. Subdural hematoma is common after acute deceleration injury from a fall or motor vehicle accident but rarely is associated with skull fracture.

CHAPTER 6

Spinal Cord

Objectives

1. Describe the structure of the adult spinal cord; compare and contrast the adult structure with the spinal cord of the newborn.
2. Describe the structure of and modalities carried by each of the major spinal cord pathways: anterolateral system; posterior columns; spinocerebellars; corticospinals.
3. Describe classic lesions of the spinal cord, including Brown-Séquard syndrome, anterior spinal artery occlusion, vitamin B_{12} neuropathy, syringomyelia, and amyotrophic lateral sclerosis.

Structure—lies within the subarachnoid space and is held in place by two pial specializations: A pair of toothed denticulate ligaments and the filum terminale (Figure 6-1).

I Gray and White Rami Communicans (Figure 6-1)

A. Gray rami communicans contain unmyelinated postganglionic sympathetic fibers. They are found at all levels of the spinal cord.

B. White rami communicans contain myelinated preganglionic sympathetic fibers. They are found from T1 to L2 (the extent of the lateral horn and the intermediolateral cell column which forms it).

II Spinal Nerves

A. 31 pairs: 8 cervical, 12 thoracic, 5 lumbar, 5 sacral, 1 coccygeal (Figures 6-1 and 6-2)

B. Contain preganglionic general visceral efferent (between T1 and L2 sympathetic and between S2 and S4 parasympathetic), general visceral afferent, general somatic efferent, and general somatic afferent fibers

C. Formed by the junction of anterior (motor) and posterior (sensory) roots, the posterior root is the site of the spinal ganglion (dorsal or posterior root ganglion), which contain all afferent cell bodies for the body (somatic and visceral)

III Conus Medullaris (Figure 6-2), the tapering inferior end of the spinal cord,

occurs in the newborn at the level of the body of the third lumbar vertebra (L3). In the adult, it occurs at the level of the inferior border of the first lumbar vertebra (L1). This is clinically relevant in determining the appropriate position for performing lumbar puncture in children and adults.

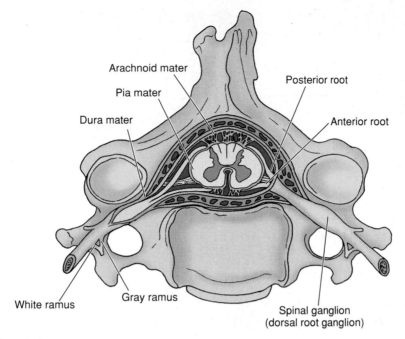

Arachnoid mater

Pia mater

Dura mater

Posterior root

Anterior root

White ramus

Gray ramus

Spinal ganglion
(dorsal root ganglion)

Figure 6-1 The spinal nerve.

IV Location of the Major Motor and Sensory Nuclei of the Spinal Cord

A. The **ciliospinal center of Budge,** from C8 to T2, contains the preganglionic sympathetic neurons that innervate the superior cervical ganglion to provide sympathetic innervation of the eye.

B. The **intermediolateral cell column,** of the lateral horn, from T1 to L2, contains all of the preganglionic sympathetic cell bodies in the body.

C. The **posterior thoracic nucleus** (nucleus dorsalis of Clarke), from C8 to L2, gives rise to the posterior spinocerebellar tract.

D. The **sacral parasympathetic nucleus,** from S2 to S4

E. The **spinal accessory nucleus,** from C1 to C6

F. The **phrenic nucleus,** from C3 to C5

G. Substantia gelatinosa and **nucleus proprius,** found at all spinal cord levels, contain neurons that mediate light touch, pain, and temperature.

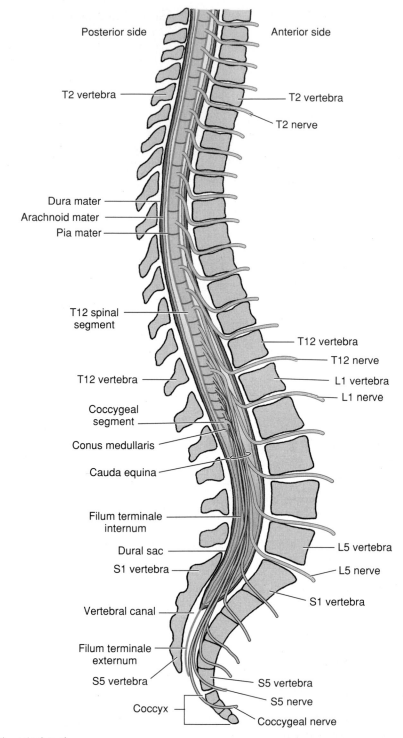

Posterior side

Anterior side

T2 vertebra

T2 vertebra

T2 nerve

Dura mater
Arachnoid mater
Pia mater

T12 spinal
segment

T12 vertebra
T12 nerve
L1 vertebra
L1 nerve

T12 vertebra

Coccygeal
segment

Conus medullaris

Cauda equina

Filum terminale
internum

Dural sac
S1 vertebra

L5 vertebra

L5 nerve

S1 vertebra

Vertebral canal

Filum terminale
externum

S5 vertebra

Coccyx

S5 vertebra

S5 nerve

Coccygeal nerve

Figure 6-2 The spinal cord.

H. Spinal Border Cells, found between L2 and S3, mediate unconscious (reflex) proprioception.

I. Somatic Motor Nuclei, found at all levels, somatotopically organized—medial group innervates more medial musculature, while the lateral group innervates appendicular musculature (Figure 6-3).

 The Cauda Equina. Anterior and posterior roots that are found in the subarachnoid space below the conus medullaris form the cauda equina.

 The Myotatic Reflex (Figure 6-4) is a monosynaptic and ipsilateral **muscle stretch reflex (MSR).** Like all reflexes, the myotatic reflex has an afferent and an efferent limb. Interruption of either limb results in **areflexia.**

A. The **afferent limb** includes a muscle spindle (receptor) and a spinal ganglion neuron and its Ia fiber.

B. The **efferent limb** includes an anterior horn motor neuron that innervates the striated muscle (effector).

C. The **five most commonly tested MSRs** are listed in Table 6-1.

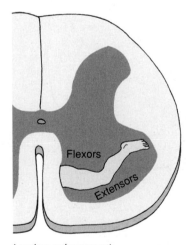

Lumbar enlargement

Figure 6-3 Somatotopic organization of the motoneurons of the anterior horn.

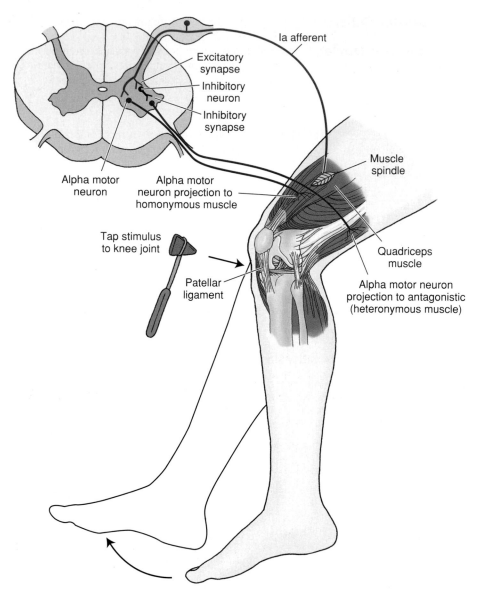

Figure 6-4 Myotatic reflex.

Table 6-1: The Five Most Commonly Tested Muscle Stretch Reflexes

Muscle Stretch Reflex	Cord Segment	Muscle
Ankle jerk	S1	Gastrocnemius
Knee jerk	L2–L4	Quadriceps
Biceps jerk	C5 and C6	Biceps brachii
Forearm jerk	C5 and C6	Brachioradialis
Triceps jerk	C7 and C8	Triceps brachii

CASE 6-1

A 46-year-old man was admitted with complaints of lower back pain that radiated down to his foot over the last 2 months. The pain was not relieved with medical therapy. What is your diagnosis?

Relevant Physical Exam Findings

- Absent right ankle jerk
- Weakness of dorsiflexion and plantar flexion
- Decreased pinprick over the dorsum of the foot

Relevant Lab Findings

- An anteroposterior myelogram demonstrated compression of the first sacral nerve root on the left at the level of the L5-S1 vertebrae.

Diagnosis

- Lumbar intervertebral disc herniation

Tracts of the Spinal Cord

 ## Posterior (Dorsal) Column—Medial Lemniscus Pathway (Figures 6-5 and 6-6)

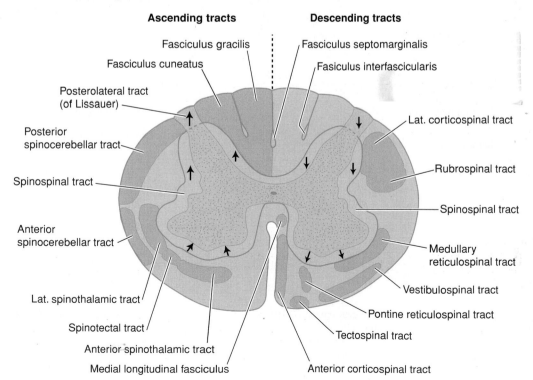

Figure 6-5 The major ascending and descending pathways of the spinal cord. The ascending tracts are shown on the left, and the descending tracts are shown on the right.

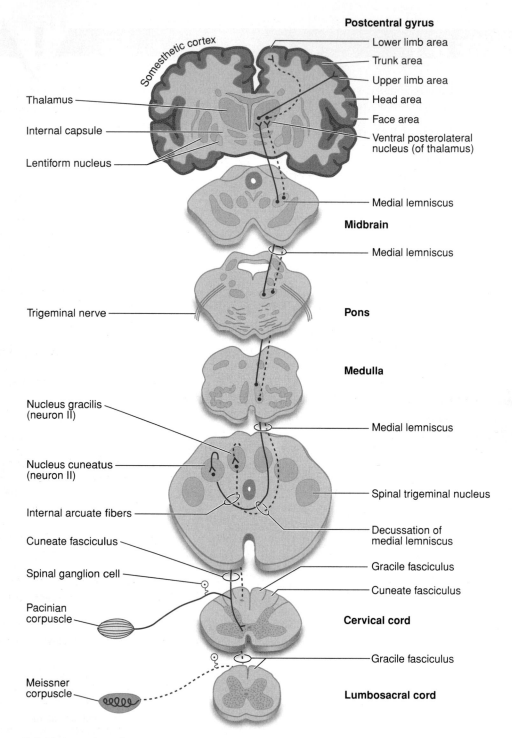

Figure 6-6 The posterior column—medial lemniscus pathway. Impulses conducted by this pathway mediate fine touch, conscious proprioception, and vibratory sense.

A. Function. The posterior column—medial lemniscus pathway mediates fine touch, conscious proprioception, and vibratory sense.

B. Receptors include Pacinian and Meissner corpuscles, joint receptors, muscle spindles, and Golgi tendon organs.

C. First-order Neurons are located in the spinal ganglia at all levels. Central processes project to the spinal cord through the medial root entry zone. First-order neurons give rise to the:
1. Gracile fasciculus from the lower extremity.
2. Cuneate fasciculus from the upper extremity.
3. Collaterals for spinal reflexes (e.g., myotatic reflex).

D. Second-order Neurons are located in the gracile and cuneate nuclei of the caudal medulla. They give rise to axons and internal arcuate fibers that decussate and form a compact fiber bundle (i.e., medial lemniscus). The medial lemniscus ascends through the contralateral brain stem and terminates in the ventral posterolateral (VPL) nucleus of the thalamus.

E. Third-order Neurons are located in the VPL nucleus of the thalamus. They project through the posterior limb of the internal capsule to the postcentral gyrus—the primary somatosensory cortex (Brodmann areas 3, 1, and 2).

F. Transection of the Posterior Column—Medial Lemniscus Tract
1. **Superior to the sensory decussation,** transection results in contralateral loss of the posterior column modalities.
2. **In the spinal cord,** transection results in ipsilateral loss of the posterior column modalities.

Anterolateral System (Figures 6-5 and 6-7)

A. Function. The anterolateral system is comprised of three main pathways: the spinothalamic tracts (lateral and medial) that mediate pain and temperature and crude touch, respectively; the spinoreticular tract, which carries pain to the reticular formation for arousal; and the spinotectal tract that mediates auditory and visual reflex orientation of the head and neck.

B. Receptors are free nerve endings. Pain ascends on both fast- and slow-conducting pain fibers (i.e., A-δ and C, respectively).

C. First-order Neurons are found in the spinal ganglia at all levels. Central projections enter the spinal cord through the posterolateral tract (of Lissauer) (lateral root entry zone) to second-order neurons.

D. Second-order Neurons are found in the posterior horn. They give rise to axons that decussate in the **anterior white commissure** and ascend in anterior aspect of the contralateral lateral funiculus. Their axons terminate in the VPL nucleus of the thalamus.

E. Third-order Neurons are found in the VPL nucleus of the thalamus. They project through the posterior limb of the internal capsule to the primary somatosensory cortex (Brodmann areas 3, 1, and 2).

F. Transection of the Lateral Spinothalamic Tract of the anterolateral system results in contralateral loss of pain and temperature inferior to the level of the lesion.

Lateral Corticospinal Tract (Figures 6-5 and 6-8)

A. Function. The lateral corticospinal tract mediates voluntary motor activity, primarily of the upper limbs.

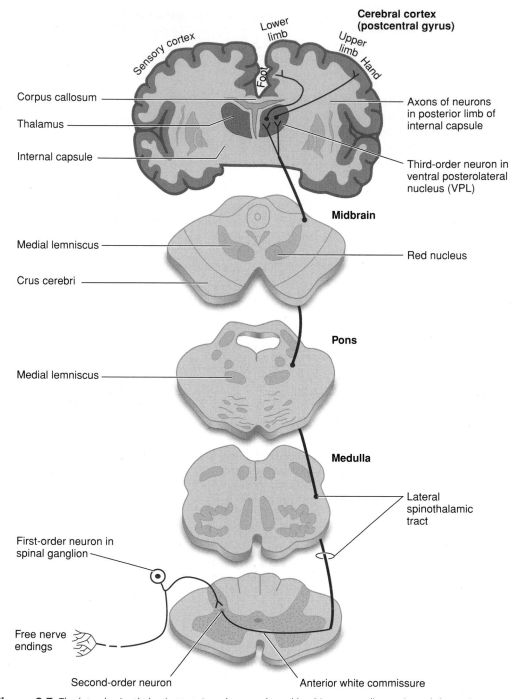

Figure 6-7 The lateral spinothalamic tract. Impulses conducted by this tract mediate pain and thermal sense.

B. Origin and Termination

1. **Origin.** The lateral corticospinal tract arises in the **premotor cortex** (Brodmann area 6) and the **primary motor cortex,** or precentral gyrus (Brodmann area 4).

2. **Termination.** The lateral corticospinal tract terminates contralaterally, through interneurons, on anterior horn motor neurons.

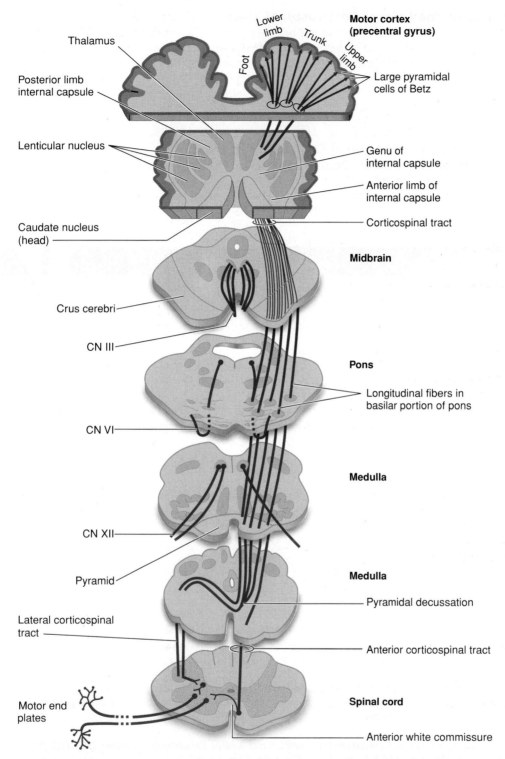

Figure 6-8 The lateral and anterior corticospinal (pyramidal) tracts. These major descending motor pathways mediate volitional motor activity.

C. Course of the Lateral Corticospinal Tract

The lateral corticospinal tract runs in the posterior limb of the internal capsule to enter the middle three-fifths of the crus cerebri of the midbrain, through the basilar pons and into the medullary pyramids. Between 85% and 90% of the corticospinal fibers cross in the pyramidal decussation as the lateral corticospinal tract, which is found in the posterior aspect of the lateral funiculus. The remaining 10% to 15% of the fibers continue as the anterior corticospinal tract. The fibers of the anterior corticospinal tract decussate in the spinal cord at the level of innervation of the lower motor neurons of the anterior horn that they innervate.

D. Transection of the Lateral Corticospinal Tract

1. **Superior to the motor decussation,** transection results in contralateral spastic paresis and Babinski sign (upward fanning of the toes).
2. **In the spinal cord,** transection results in ipsilateral spastic paresis and Babinski sign.

CASE 6-2

A 17-year-old man complained of pain on the left side of his chest and progressive weakness of his left lower limb for 2 months before coming to the clinic. What is the most likely diagnosis?

Relevant Physical Exam Findings

● Neurologic evaluation revealed weakness in the left lower limb; spasticity and hyperreflexia at the knee and ankle were also observed.
● On the left side, a loss of two-point discrimination, vibratory sense, and conscious proprioception below the hip was observed. A loss of pain and temperature sensation below the T7 dermatome was observed on the right side.

Diagnosis

● Brown-Séquard syndrome, resulting from an upper motor neuron lesion at T5-T6 spinal cord levels, represents an incomplete spinal cord lesion characterized by symptoms indicative of hemisection of the spinal cord. It involves ipsilateral hemiplegia with contralateral pain and temperature deficits.

Diseases of the Motor Neurons and Corticospinal Tracts (Figures 6-9 and 6-10)

A. Upper Motor Neuron (UMN) Lesions are caused by lesions of the corticospinal tract or destruction of the cortical cells of origin. UMN lesions result in spastic paresis with pyramidal signs (Babinski sign) and hyperreflexia.

B. Lower Motor Neuron (LMN) Lesions are caused by damage to the motor neurons. They result in flaccid paralysis, hyporeflexia, atrophy, fasciculations, and fibrillations. **Poliomyelitis or Werdnig–Hoffmann disease** (Figure 6-10A) results from damage to motor neurons.

C. An Example of a Combined UMN and LMN Disease is Amyotrophic Lateral Sclerosis (ALS, or Lou Gehrig Disease) (Figure 6-10D). ALS is caused by damage to the corticospinal tracts, with pyramidal signs, and by damage to the LMNs, with LMN symptoms. Patients with ALS have no sensory deficits.

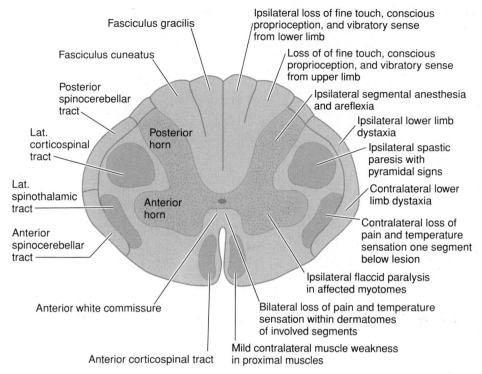

Fasciculus gracilis

Ipsilateral loss of fine touch, conscious proprioception, and vibratory sense from lower limb

Fasciculus cuneatus

Loss of of fine touch, conscious proprioception, and vibratory sense from upper limb

Posterior spinocerebellar tract

Ipsilateral segmental anesthesia and areflexia

Posterior horn

Ipsilateral lower limb dystaxia

Lat. corticospinal tract

Ipsilateral spastic paresis with pyramidal signs

Lat. spinothalamic tract

Anterior horn

Contralateral lower limb dystaxia

Anterior spinocerebellar tract

Contralateral loss of pain and temperature sensation one segment below lesion

Anterior white commissure

Ipsilateral flaccid paralysis in affected myotomes

Bilateral loss of pain and temperature sensation within dermatomes of involved segments

Anterior corticospinal tract

Mild contralateral muscle weakness in proximal muscles

Figure 6-9 Transverse section of the cervical spinal cord. The clinically important ascending and descending pathways are shown on the left. Clinical deficits that result from the interruption of these pathways are shown on the right.

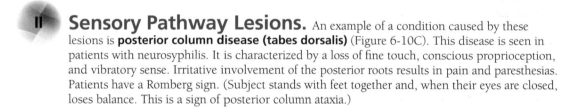

II   Sensory Pathway Lesions. An example of a condition caused by these lesions is **posterior column disease (tabes dorsalis)** (Figure 6-10C). This disease is seen in patients with neurosyphilis. It is characterized by a loss of fine touch, conscious proprioception, and vibratory sense. Irritative involvement of the posterior roots results in pain and paresthesias. Patients have a Romberg sign. (Subject stands with feet together and, when their eyes are closed, loses balance. This is a sign of posterior column ataxia.)

III   Combined Motor and Sensory Lesions

A. Spinal Cord Hemisection (Brown-Séquard Syndrome) (Figure 6-10E) is caused by damage to the following structures:
1. **Posterior columns (gracile [leg] and cuneate [arm] fasciculi).** Damage results in ipsilateral loss of fine touch, conscious proprioception, and vibratory sense.
2. **Lateral corticospinal tract.** Damage results in ipsilateral spastic paresis with pyramidal signs inferior to the lesion.
3. **Lateral spinothalamic tract.** Damage results in contralateral loss of pain and temperature sensation one to two segments inferior to the lesion.
4. **Hypothalamospinal tract.** Damage results in ipsilateral Horner syndrome (i.e., miosis, ptosis, hemianhidrosis, and apparent enophthalmos).
5. **Anterior horn.** Damage results in ipsilateral flaccid paralysis.

B. Anterior Spinal Artery Occlusion (Figure 6-10F) causes infarction of the anterior two-thirds of the spinal cord but spares the posterior columns and horns. It results in damage to the following structures:

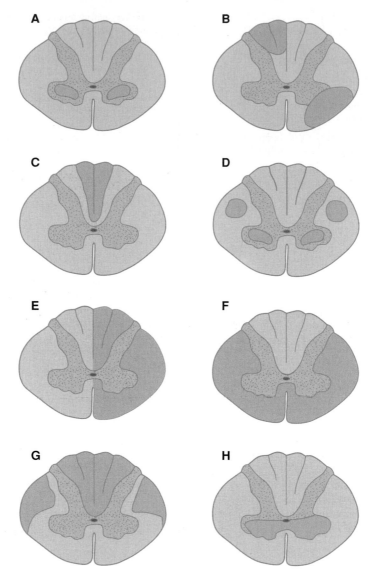

Figure 6-10 Classic lesions of the spinal cord. **A.** Poliomyelitis and progressive infantile muscular atrophy (Werdnig–Hoffmann disease). **B.** Multiple sclerosis. **C.** Posterior column disease (tabes dorsalis). **D.** Amyotrophic lateral sclerosis. **E.** Hemisection of the spinal cord (Brown-Séquard syndrome). **F.** Complete anterior spinal artery occlusion. **G.** Subacute combined degeneration (vitamin B$_{12}$ neuropathy). **H.** Syringomyelia.

1. **Lateral corticospinal tracts.** Damage results in bilateral spastic paresis with pyramidal signs inferior to the lesion.
2. **Lateral spinothalamic tracts.** Damage results in bilateral loss of pain and temperature sensation inferior to the lesion.
3. **Hypothalamospinal tract.** Damage results in bilateral Horner syndrome.
4. **Anterior horns.** Damage results in bilateral flaccid paralysis.
5. **Corticospinal tracts to the sacral parasympathetic centers at S2-S4.** Damage results in loss of voluntary bladder and bowel control.

C. Subacute Combined Degeneration (Vitamin B$_{12}$ Neuropathy) (Figure 6-10G)

is caused by pernicious (megaloblastic) anemia. It results from damage to the following structures:

1. **Posterior columns (gracile and cuneate fasciculi).** Damage results in bilateral loss of fine touch, conscious proprioception, and vibratory sense.

2. **Lateral corticospinal tracts.** Damage results in bilateral spastic paresis with pyramidal signs.

3. **Spinocerebellar tracts.** Damage results in bilateral arm and leg dystaxia.

D. Syringomyelia (Figure 6-10H) is a central cavitation of the spinal cord, resulting from a congenital defect, trauma, hemorrhage, or infection. Expansion of the syrinx may result in damage to nearby structures, including:

1. **Anterior white commissure.** Damage to decussating lateral spinothalamic axons causes bilateral loss of pain and temperature sensation.

2. **Anterior horns.** LMN lesions result in flaccid paralysis, hyperreflexia and wasting of the affected musculature.

E. Friedreich Ataxia—has the same spinal cord pathology and symptoms as subacute combined degeneration.

F. Multiple Sclerosis (Figure 6-10B), demyelination primarily involves the white matter of the spinal cord. Damage is random and asymmetric.

 Peripheral Nervous System (PNS) Lesions. An example of a PNS lesion is **Guillain–Barré syndrome** (acute idiopathic polyneuritis, or postinfectious polyneuritis). It primarily affects the motor fibers of the anterior roots and peripheral nerves, and it produces LMN symptoms (i.e., muscle weakness, flaccid paralysis, and hyporeflexia). Guillain–Barré syndrome has the following features:

A. Demyelination and edema.

B. Upper cervical root (C4) involvement and respiratory paralysis are common.

C. Caudal cranial nerve involvement with facial diplegia is present in 50% of cases.

D. Elevated protein levels may cause papilledema.

E. Sensory fibers may be affected, resulting in paresthesias.

F. The protein level in the cerebrospinal fluid is elevated but without pleocytosis **(albuminocytologic dissociation).**

 Intervertebral Disk Herniation is seen at the L4 to L5 or L5 to S1 interspace in 90% of cases. It appears at the C5 to C6 or C6 to C7 interspace in 10% of cases.

A. Intervertebral disk herniation consists of prolapse, or herniation, of the **nucleus pulposus through the defective anulus fibrosus and into the vertebral canal.**

B. The nucleus pulposus **impinges on the spinal roots,** resulting in spinal root symptoms (i.e., paresthesias, pain, sensory loss, hyporeflexia, and muscle weakness).

 Cauda Equina Syndrome (Spinal Roots L3 to C0) may result from a nerve root tumor, an ependymoma, a dermoid tumor, or from a lipoma of the terminal spinal cord. It is characterized by:

A. Severe radicular unilateral pain.

B. Sensory distribution in a unilateral **saddle-shaped** area.

C. Unilateral muscle atrophy and absent quadriceps (L3) and ankle jerk (S1) reflex activity.

D. Unremarkable incontinence and sexual function.

E. Gradual and unilateral onset.

VII Conus Medullaris Syndrome (Cord Segments S3 to C0)

usually results from an intramedullary tumor (e.g., ependymoma). It is characterized by:

A. Pain, usually bilateral and not severe.

B. Sensory distribution in a bilateral **saddle-shaped** area.

C. Unremarkable muscle changes; normal quadriceps and ankle jerk reflexes.

D. Severely impaired incontinence and sexual function.

E. Sudden and bilateral onset.

CHAPTER 7

Brainstem

Objectives

1. Identify the brainstem nuclei associated with the cranial nerves and be able to locate them on a brainstem cross section.
2. Identify the cranial nerves where they connect to the brainstem.
3. Describe the reticular formation—connections, functions, and structure.
4. Describe the result of occlusion of the anterior spinal artery and the posterior inferior cerebellar artery, include all brainstem nuclei and pathways affected.
5. Describe medial longitudinal fasciculus syndrome and Weber syndrome.

Introduction. The brainstem includes the **medulla, pons,** and **midbrain.** It extends from the pyramidal decussation inferiorly to the posterior commissure superiorly. The brainstem receives its blood supply from the vertebrobasilar system. It gives rise to CNs III to X and XII (Figures 7-1 and 7-2).

Cross Section Through the Caudal Medulla (Figure 7-3)

1. **Pyramid** (corticospinal fibers)
2. **Nucleus gracilis and nucleus cuneatus**—give rise to **arcuate fibers** that cross the midline to form the **medial lemniscus**
3. **Anterior** and **posterior spinocerebellar tracts**
4. **Inferior olivary nucleus**
5. **Accessory cuneate nucleus**

Cross Section Through the Mid-Medulla (Figure 7-4)

1. **Hypoglossal nucleus**
2. **Dorsal motor nucleus of the vagus**—preganglionic parasympathetic cell bodies that send fibers into CN X
3. **Solitary nucleus**—special sense nucleus
4. **Medial longitudinal fasciculus**—yolks together cranial nerve nuclei from opposite sides of the brainstem
5. **Tectospinal tract**—fibers descending from the midbrain colliculi to lower motor neurons of the cervical spinal cord

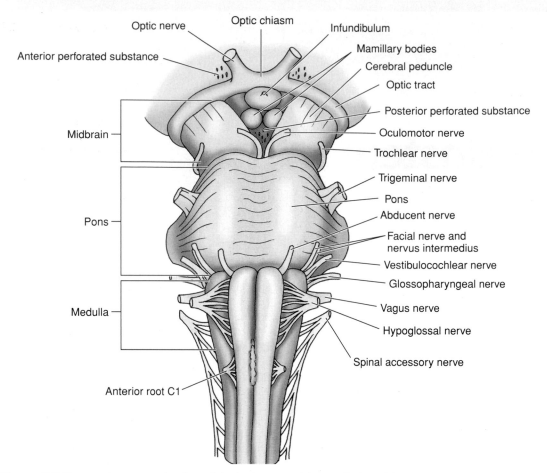

Figure 7-1 The anterior or ventral surface of the brainstem and the attached cranial nerves.

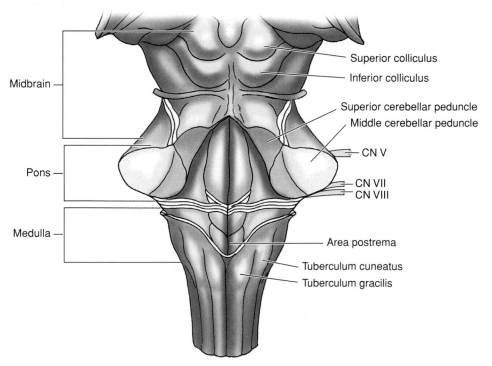

Figure 7-2 The posterior or dorsal surface of the brainstem.

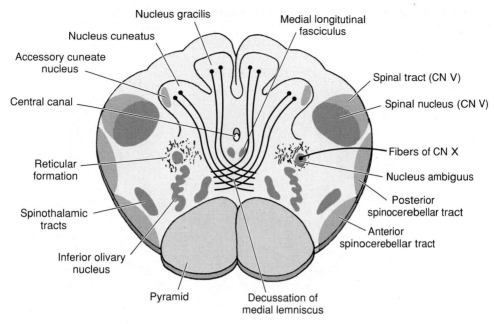

Figure 7-3 Caudal medulla.

6. **Nucleus ambiguus**—lower motor neuron nucleus that sends fibers into CNs IX and X
7. **Medial lemniscus**
8. **Inferior cerebellar peduncle**

 IV **Cross Section Through the Rostral Medulla** (Figure 7-5)

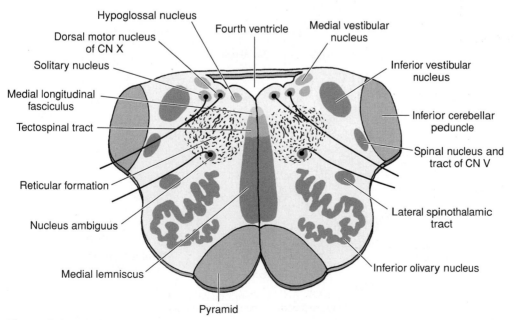

Figure 7-4 Mid-medulla.

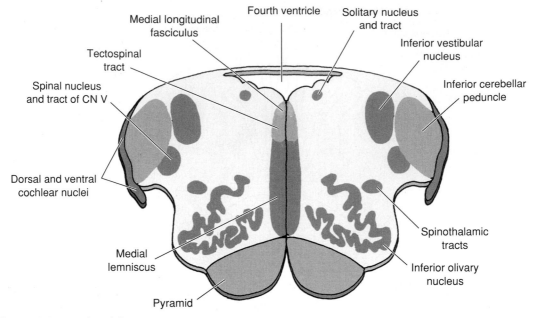

Figure 7-5 Rostral medulla.

1. **Spinothalamic tracts** (spinal lemniscus)
2. **Spinal nucleus** and **tract of trigeminal nerve**
3. **Inferior cerebellar peduncle**—contains olivocerebellar, cuneocerebellar, and posterior spinocerebellar tracts

 Cross Section Through the Caudal Pons (Figure 7-6). The pons has a posterior tegmentum and an anterior base.

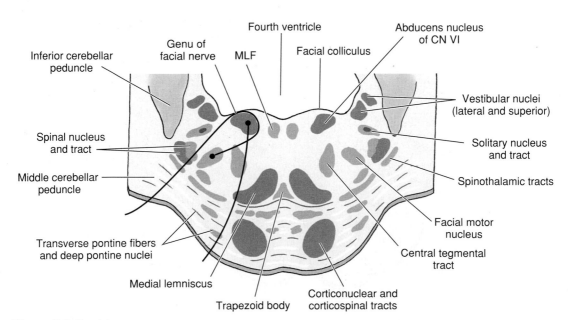

Figure 7-6 Caudal pons.

1. **Medial longitudinal fasciculus** (MLF)
2. **Abducent nucleus of CN VI** (underlies facial colliculus)
3. **Genu (internal) of CN VII** (underlies facial nerve; facial colliculus)
4. **Medial lemniscus**
5. **Corticospinal and corticonuclear tracts** (in the base of the pons)
6. **Facial motor nucleus** (CN VII)
7. **Spinal nucleus and tract of trigeminal nerve** (CN V)
8. **Spinothalamic tracts** (spinal lemniscus)
9. **Vestibular nuclei of CN VIII**
10. **Inferior and middle cerebellar peduncle**
11. **Central tegmental tract**—fiber pathway traversing the reticular formation

 ## Cross Section Through the Mid-Pons (Figure 7-7)

1. **Raphe nuclei**
2. **Deep pontine nuclei** and **transverse pontine fibers**
3. **Superior cerebellar peduncle**—main cerebellar outflow pathway, also contains decussating anterior spinocerebellar fibers

 ## Cross Section Through the Rostral Pons (Figure 7-8)

1. **Mesencephalic nucleus**—unconscious proprioception for the head
2. **Locus ceruleus**—source of norepinephrine for the brain
3. **Cerebral aqueduct**—connects the third and fourth ventricles
4. **Periaqueductal gray**—involved in pain modulation, source of serotonin

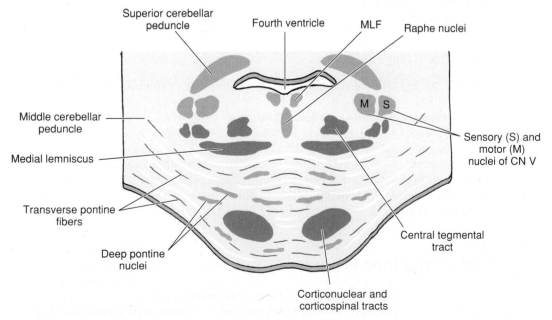

Figure 7-7 Mid-pons.

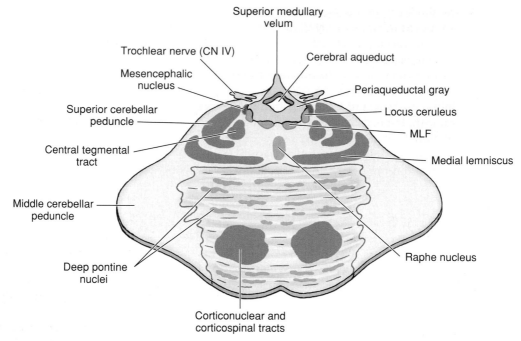

Figure 7-8 Rostral pons.

VIII Cross Section Through the Caudal Midbrain (Figure 7-9).

The midbrain has a posterior tectum, an intermediate tegmentum, and a base. The cerebral aqueduct lies between the tectum and the tegmentum.

Medial lemniscus
1. **Inferior colliculus**—auditory relay nucleus
2. **Trochlear nucleus**—lower motor neuron nucleus that innervates the superior oblique
3. **Cerebral aqueduct**
4. **Crus cerebri** (basis pedunculi cerebri or cerebral peduncle)—composed of descending fibers.

IX Cross Section Through the Rostral Medulla (Figure 7-10)

1. **Superior colliculus**—visual relay nucleus
2. **Oculomotor nucleus**—lower motor neuron nucleus that innervates the majority of the extraocular musculature
3. **Red nucleus**—part of the primitive motor system, involved in coordination
4. **Ventral tegmental area**—source of dopamine, involved in the reward system
5. **Spinothalamic** and **trigeminothalamic tracts**
6. **Medial lemniscus**

X Corticonuclear Fibers project bilaterally to all motor cranial nerve nuclei except

the facial nucleus. The division of the facial nerve nucleus that innervates the **upper face** (the orbicularis oculi and above) **receives bilateral corticonuclear input.** The division of the facial nerve nucleus that innervates the **lower face receives** only **contralateral corticonuclear input.**

Lesions of the Brainstem

 Lesions of the Medulla (Figure 7-6)

A. Medial Medullary Syndrome (Anterior Spinal Artery Syndrome). Affected structures include the following:

1. **Corticospinal tract** (medullary pyramid). Lesions result in contralateral spastic hemiparesis;
2. **Medial lemniscus.** Lesions result in contralateral loss of tactile and vibration sensation from the trunk and extremities;
3. **Hypoglossal nucleus** and its intra-axial fibers. Lesions result in ipsilateral flaccid hemiparalysis of the tongue. When protruded, the tongue points to the side of the lesion (i.e., the weak side). See Figure 9.8.

B. Lateral Medullary (Wallenberg; Posterior Inferior Cerebellar Artery [PICA]) Syndrome is characterized by dissociated sensory loss. Affected structures include the following:

1. **Vestibular nuclei.** Lesions result in nystagmus, nausea, vomiting, and vertigo;
2. **Inferior cerebellar peduncle.** Lesions result in ipsilateral cerebellar signs (e.g., dystaxia, dysmetria [past pointing], and dysdiadochokinesia);
3. **Nucleus ambiguus.** Lesions result in ipsilateral laryngeal, pharyngeal, and palatal hemiparalysis (i.e., loss of the gag reflex [efferent limb], dysarthria, dysphagia, and dysphonia [hoarseness]);
4. **Glossopharyngeal nerve roots.** Lesions result in loss of the gag reflex (afferent limb);
5. **Vagal nerve roots.** Lesions result in the same deficits as seen in lesions involving the nucleus ambiguus;
6. **Spinothalamic tracts (spinal lemniscus).** Lesions result in contralateral loss of pain and temperature sensation;
7. **Spinal trigeminal nucleus and tract.** Lesions result in ipsilateral loss of pain and temperature sensation from the face (facial hemianesthesia);
8. **Descending sympathetic tract.** Lesions result in ipsilateral Horner syndrome (i.e., ptosis, miosis, hemianhidrosis, and apparent enophthalmos).

 Lesions of the Pons (Figure 7-7A)

A. Medial Inferior Pontine Syndrome results from occlusion of the paramedian branches of the basilar artery. Affected structures include the following:

1. **Corticospinal tract.** Lesions result in contralateral spastic hemiparesis.
2. **Medial lemniscus.** Lesions result in contralateral loss of tactile sensation from the trunk and extremities.
3. **Abducent nerve roots.** Lesions result in ipsilateral lateral rectus paralysis.

B. Lateral Inferior Pontine Syndrome (anterior inferior cerebellar artery syndrome; Figure 7-7B). Affected structures include the following:

1. **Facial nucleus** and intra-axial nerve fibers. Lesions result in:
   a. Ipsilateral facial paralysis;
   b. Ipsilateral loss of taste from the anterior two-thirds of the tongue;
   c. Ipsilateral loss of lacrimation and reduced salivation;
   d. Loss of the efferent limb of the corneal blink and stapedial reflexes (hyperacusis).
2. **Cochlear nuclei** and intra-axial nerve fibers. Lesions result in ipsilateral deafness;
3. **Vestibular nuclei** and intra-axial nerve fibers. Lesions result in nystagmus, nausea, vomiting, and vertigo;

4. **Spinal nucleus and tract of the trigeminal nerve.** Lesions result in ipsilateral loss of pain and temperature sensation from the face (facial hemianesthesia);
5. **Middle and inferior cerebellar peduncles.** Lesions result in ipsilateral limb and gait dystaxia;
6. **Spinothalamic tracts (spinal lemniscus).** Lesions result in contralateral loss of pain and temperature sensation from the trunk and extremities;
7. **Descending sympathetic tract.** Lesions result in ipsilateral Horner syndrome.

C. **MLF Syndrome (Internuclear Ophthalmoplegia)** **(Figure 7-7C)** interrupts fibers from the contralateral abducent nucleus that project through the MLF to the ipsilateral medial rectus subnucleus of CN III. It causes **medial rectus palsy** on attempted lateral conjugate gaze and **nystagmus** in the abducting eye. Convergence remains intact. This syndrome is often seen in patients with **multiple sclerosis.**

D. **Facial Colliculus Syndrome** usually results from a pontine glioma or a vascular accident. The internal genu of CN VII and the abducent nucleus underlie the facial colliculus.
1. Lesions of the **internal genu** of the **facial nerve** cause:
   a. Ipsilateral facial paralysis;
   b. Ipsilateral loss of the corneal blink reflex (efferent limb).
2. Lesions of the **abducent nucleus** cause:
   a. Lateral rectus paralysis (medial strabismus);
   b. Horizontal diplopia.

 III **Lesions of the Midbrain** (Figure 7-8)

A. **Posterior Midbrain (Parinaud) Syndrome** **(see Figure 7-8A)** is often the result of a pinealoma or germinoma of the pineal region. Affected structures include the following:
1. **Superior colliculus** and **pretectal area.** Lesions cause paralysis of upward and downward gaze, pupillary disturbances, and absence of convergence;
2. **Cerebral aqueduct.** Compression causes noncommunicating hydrocephalus.

B. **Paramedian Midbrain (Benedikt) Syndrome** **(see Figure 7-8B).** Affected structures include the following:
1. **Oculomotor nerve roots** (intra-axial fibers). Lesions cause complete ipsilateral oculomotor paralysis. Eye abduction and depression is caused by the intact lateral rectus (CN VI) and superior oblique (CN IV). Ptosis (paralysis of the levator palpebrae superioris) and fixation and dilation of the ipsilateral pupil (complete internal ophthalmoplegia) also occur;
2. **Dentatothalamic fibers.** Lesions cause contralateral cerebellar dystaxia with intention tremor;
3. **Medial lemniscus.** Lesions result in contralateral loss of tactile sensation from the trunk and extremities.

C. **Medial Midbrain (Weber) Syndrome** **(see Figure 7-8C).** Affected structures and resultant deficits include the following:
1. **Oculomotor nerve roots** (intra-axial fibers). Lesions cause complete ipsilateral oculomotor paralysis. Eye abduction and depression are caused by intact lateral rectus (CN VI) and superior oblique (CN IV). Ptosis, fixation, and dilation of the ipsilateral pupil also occur;
2. **Corticospinal tracts.** Lesions result in contralateral spastic hemiparesis;
3. **Corticonuclear fibers.** Lesions cause contralateral weakness of the lower face (CN VII), tongue (CN XII), and palate (CN X). The upper face division of the facial nucleus receives bilateral corticonuclear input. The uvula and pharyngeal wall are pulled toward the normal side (CN X), and the protruded tongue points to the weak side.

IV **Acoustic Neuroma (Schwannoma)** (Figure 7-9) is a benign tumor of Schwann cells that affects the vestibulocochlear nerve (CN VIII). It accounts for 8% of all intracranial tumors. It is a posterior fossa tumor near the internal auditory meatus and cerebellopontine angle. The neuroma often compresses the facial nerve (CN VII), which accompanies CN VIII in the cerebellopontine angle and internal auditory meatus. It may impinge on the pons and affect the spinal trigeminal tract (CN V). **Schwannomas** occur twice as often in women as in men. Affected structures and resultant deficits include the following:

A. Cochlear Division of CN VIII. Damage results in tinnitus and unilateral nerve deafness;

B. Vestibular Division of CN VIII. Damage results in vertigo, nystagmus, nausea, vomiting, and unsteadiness of gait;

C. Facial Nerve (CN VII). Damage results in facial weakness and loss of the corneal blink reflex (efferent limb);

D. Spinal Tract of Trigeminal Nerve (CN V). Damage results in paresthesia, anesthesia of the ipsilateral face, and loss of the corneal blink reflex (afferent limb).
NEUROFIBROMATOSIS TYPE 2. This disorder often occurs with bilateral acoustic neuromas.

 V **Jugular Foramen Syndrome** usually results from a posterior fossa tumor (e.g., **glomus jugulare tumor,** the most common inner ear tumor) that compresses CNs IX, X, and XI. Affected structures and resultant deficits include the following:

A. Glossopharyngeal Nerve (CN IX). Damage results in:
   1. Ipsilateral loss of the gag reflex;
   2. Ipsilateral loss of pain, temperature, and taste in the tongue.

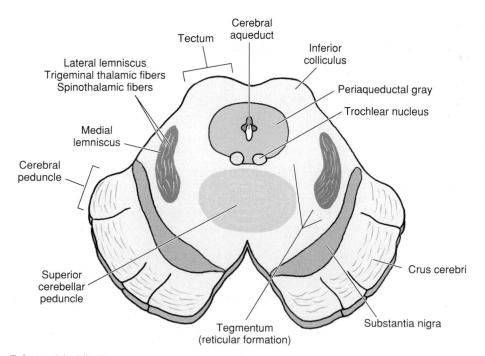

Figure 7-9 Caudal midbrain.

B. Vagal Nerve (CN X). Damage results in:
1. Ipsilateral paralysis of the soft palate and larynx;
2. Ipsilateral loss of the gag reflex.

C. Accessory Nerve (CN XI). Damage results in:
1. Paralysis of sternocleidomastoid, which results in the inability to turn the head to the opposite side;
2. Paralysis of trapezius, which causes shoulder droop and inability to shrug the shoulder.

 "Locked-in" Syndrome is a lesion of the base of the pons as the result of infarction, trauma, tumor, or demyelination. The corticospinal and corticonuclear tracts are affected bilaterally. The oculomotor and trochlear nerves are not injured. Patients are conscious and may communicate through vertical eye movements.

 Central Pontine Myelinolysis is a lesion of the base of the pons that affects the corticospinal and corticonuclear tracts. More than 75% of cases are associated with alcoholism or rapid correction of hyponatremia. Symptoms include spastic quadriparesis, pseudobulbar palsy, and mental changes. This condition may become the locked-in syndrome.

 "Top of the Basilar" Syndrome results from embolic occlusion of the rostral basilar artery. Neurologic signs include optic ataxia and psychic paralysis of fixation of gaze **(Balint syndrome),** ectopic pupils, somnolence, and cortical blindness, with or without visual anosognosia **(Anton syndrome).**

 Subclavian Steal Syndrome (Figure 7-10) results from thrombosis of the left subclavian artery proximal to the vertebral artery. Blood is shunted in the left vertebral artery and into the left subclavian artery. Clinical signs include transient weakness and claudication of the left upper limb on exercise and vertebrobasilar insufficiency (i.e., vertigo, dizziness).

 The Cerebellopontine Angle is the junction of the medulla, pons, and cerebellum. CNs VII and VIII are found there. Five brain tumors, including a cyst, are often located in the cerebellopontine angle cistern. Remember the acronym **SAME: s**chwannoma **(75%), a**rachnoid cyst **(1%), m**eningioma **(10%),** and **e**pendymoma **(1%)** and **e**pidermoid **(5%).** The percentages refer to cerebellopontine angle tumors.

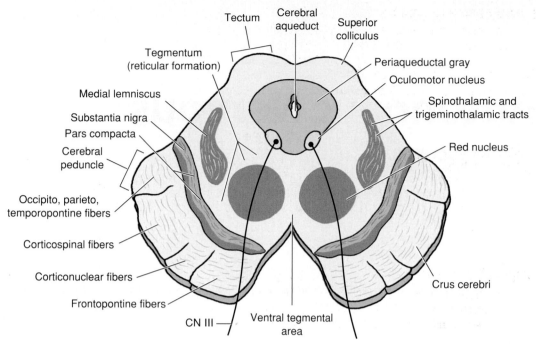

Figure 7-10 Rostral midbrain.

CASE 7-1

For several weeks, a 60-year-old hypertensive, diabetic man has experienced sudden dizziness, facial pain, double vision, and difficulty in walking. He is also having problems in swallowing and speaking. What is the most likely diagnosis?

Relevant Physical Exam Findings

- Decreased temperature and pain sense below the left T-4 level
- Horner syndrome on the right side
- Decreased position sensation in the right fingers and toes
- Ataxia and mild weakness in the right limbs

Relevant Lab Finding

- An infarct involving the right lateral part of the lower medulla and the cerebellum seen on brain magnetic resonance image.

Diagnosis

- Wallenberg's syndrome is an infarction involving the lateral or medial branches of the posterior inferior cerebellar artery.

CHAPTER 8

Autonomic Nervous System

Objectives

1. List the functions of the sympathetic and parasympathetic divisions of the autonomic nervous system (ANS), using Table 8.1 as a reference.
2. Describe the location(s) of the pre- and postganglionic cell bodies of the sympathetic and parasympathetic divisions of the ANS.
3. Trace the pathways that pre- and postganglionic fibers take to reach their destinations.

 Introduction. The autonomic nervous system (ANS) is a general visceral efferent motor system that **controls and regulates smooth muscle, cardiac muscle, and glands.**

A. The ANS consists of a two-neuron chain from the CNS to the effector: a pre- and postganglionic neuron.

B. Autonomic Output is generally reflexive and is influenced rostrally by the **hypothalamus.**

C. The ANS has **three divisions:**

1. **Sympathetic (Figure 8-1).**
   - Prepares the body for action—fight or flight
   - Uses a lot of energy, as it upregulates function in a nonspecific way
   - Preganglionic cell bodies in the spinal cord between T1 and L2, form the intermediolateral cell column of the lateral horn.
   - Postganglionic cell bodies are found in the **sympathetic chain**—primarily for innervation of the body wall (i.e., erector pili, blood vessels, and sweat glands) or in **prevertebral ganglia** for innervation of the gut.

2. **Parasympathetic (Figure 8-2).**
   - Responsible for resting state of the body—rest and digest
   - Conserves energy, functions more specifically because of the short postganglionic fibers (i.e., it can activate targets with more specificity)
   - Preganglionic cell bodies in the brainstem—associated with CNs III, VII, IX, and X, and the sacral spinal cord S2-S4
   - Postganglionic cell bodies are found in the ciliary, otic, pterygopalatine, or submandibular ganglia for the head—all postganglionic parasympathetic fibers in the head run in branches of CN V to reach their targets, and in the walls of the target organ for the body.

3. **Enteric.** The enteric nervous system is composed of the intramural ganglia of the gastrointestinal tract, submucosal plexus, and myenteric plexus.

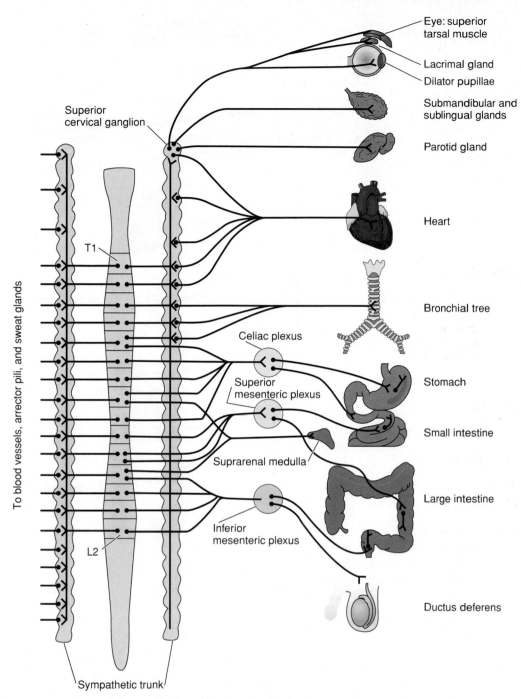

Figure 8-1 The sympathetic (thoracolumbar) innervation of the autonomic nervous system.

Cranial Nerves (CN) With Parasympathetic Components include the following:

A. CN III—preganglionic cell bodies in the **accessory oculomotor (Edinger–Westphal)** nucleus; postganglionic cell bodies in the **ciliary ganglion.**

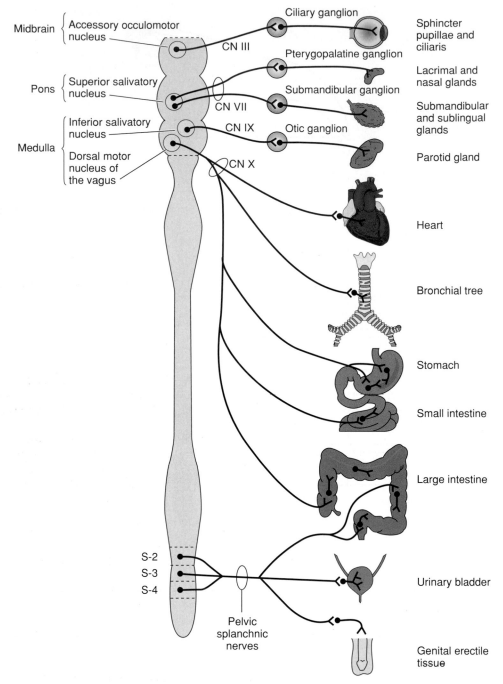

Figure 8-2 The parasympathetic (craniosacral) innervation of the autonomic nervous system.

B. CN VII—preganglionic cell bodies in the **superior salivatory nucleus;** postganglionic cell bodies in the **pterygopalatine** and **submandibular ganglia.**

C. CN IX—preganglionic cell bodies in the **inferior salivatory nucleus;** postganglionic cell bodies in the **otic ganglion.**

D. CN X—preganglionic cell bodies in the **dorsal motor nucleus of the vagus;** postganglionic cell bodies in **intramural ganglia.**

Communicating Rami include the following:

A. White Rami Communicantes, which are found between T-1 and L-2 and are myelinated. Carry visceral afferents and preganglionic sympathetic fibers to the sympathetic chain.

B. Gray Rami Communicantes, which are found at all spinal levels and are unmyelinated. Carry postganglionic sympathetic fibers to the spinal nerve.

 Neurotransmitters of the ANS include the following:

A. Acetylcholine, which is the neurotransmitter of the preganglionic neurons, as well as the postganglionic parasympathetics.

B. Norepinephrine, which is the neurotransmitter of the postganglionic sympathetic neurons.

C. Dopamine, which is the neurotransmitter of the small, intensely fluorescent (SIF) cells, which are interneurons of the sympathetic ganglia.

 Clinical Correlation

A. Megacolon (Hirschsprung Disease or Congenital Aganglionic Megacolon) is characterized by extreme dilation and hypertrophy of the colon, with fecal retention, and by the absence of ganglion cells in the myenteric plexus. It occurs when neural crest cells do not migrate into the colon.

B. Familial Dysautonomia (Riley–Day Syndrome) predominantly affects Jewish children. It is an autosomal recessive trait that is characterized by abnormal sweating, unstable blood pressure (e.g., orthostatic hypotension), difficulty in feeding (as a result of inadequate muscle tone in the gastrointestinal tract), and progressive sensory loss. It results in the loss of neurons in the autonomic and sensory ganglia.

C. Raynaud Disease is a painful disorder of the terminal arteries of the extremities. It is characterized by idiopathic paroxysmal bilateral cyanosis of the digits (as a result of arterial and arteriolar constriction because of cold or emotion). It may be treated by preganglionic sympathectomy.

D. Peptic Ulcer Disease results from excessive production of hydrochloric acid because of increased parasympathetic (tone) stimulation.

E. Horner Syndrome (see Chapter 14) is oculosympathetic paralysis. Characterized by ptosis, anhidrosis, miosis, and enophthalmos.

F. Shy–Drager Syndrome involves preganglionic sympathetic neurons. It is characterized by orthostatic hypotension, anhidrosis, impotence, and bladder atonicity.

G. Botulism. The toxin of *Clostridium botulinum* blocks the release of acetylcholine and results in paralysis of striated muscles. Autonomic effects include dry eyes, dry mouth, and gastrointestinal ileus (bowel obstruction).

H. Lambert–Eaton Myasthenic Syndrome is a preganglionic disorder of neuromuscular transmission in which acetylcholine release is impaired, resulting in autonomic dysfunction (such as dry mouth) as well as proximal muscle weakness and abnormal tendon reflexes.

Table 8-1: Sympathetic and Parasympathetic Activity on Organ Systems

Structure	Sympathetic Function	Parasympathetic Function
Eye		
Radial muscle of iris	Dilation of pupil (mydriasis)	
Circular muscle of iris		Constriction of pupil (miosis)
Ciliary muscle of ciliary body		Contraction for near vision
Lacrimal glands		Stimulation of secretion
Salivary glands	Viscous secretion	Watery secretion
Sweat glands		
Thermoregulatory	Increase	
Apocrine (stress)	Increase	
Heart		
Sinoatrial node	Acceleration	Deceleration (vagal arrest)
Atrioventricular node	Increase in conduction velocity	Decrease in conduction velocity
Contractility	Increase	Decrease (atria)
Vascular smooth muscle		
Skin, splanchnic vessels	Contraction	
Skeletal muscle vessels	Relaxation	
Bronchiolar smooth muscle	Relaxation	Contraction
Gastrointestinal tract		
Smooth muscle		
Walls	Relaxation	Contraction
Sphincters	Contraction	Relaxation
Secretions and motility	Decrease	Increase
Genitourinary tract		
Smooth muscle		
Bladder wall	Little or no effect	Contraction
Sphincter	Contraction	Relaxation
Penis, seminal vesicles	Ejaculation[a]	Erection[a]
Adrenal medulla	Secretion of epinephrine and norepinephrine	
Metabolic functions		
Liver	Gluconeogenesis and glycogenolysis	
Fat cells	Lipolysis	
Kidney	Renin release	

[a]Note erection versus ejaculation: Remember point and shoot, where *p,* parasympathetic; *s,* sympathetic.
Reprinted from Fix J. *BRS Neuroanatomy*. Media, PA: Williams & Wilkins; 1991, with permission.

CHAPTER 9

Cranial Nerves

Objectives

1. List the cranial nerves by name and number, including the characteristic fiber types and functions of each (see table in Appendix I for summary).
2. Trace the pathway of each cranial nerve from brainstem to target organ, including relevant nuclei and bony foramina through which each travels.
3. Outline the effects of lesioning each cranial nerve at key points along its course.

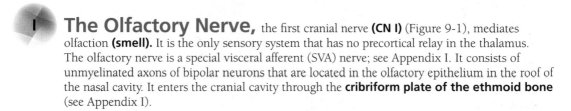

I **The Olfactory Nerve,** the first cranial nerve **(CN I)** (Figure 9-1), mediates olfaction **(smell).** It is the only sensory system that has no precortical relay in the thalamus. The olfactory nerve is a special visceral afferent (SVA) nerve; see Appendix I. It consists of unmyelinated axons of bipolar neurons that are located in the olfactory epithelium in the roof of the nasal cavity. It enters the cranial cavity through the **cribriform plate of the ethmoid bone** (see Appendix I).

A. Olfactory Pathway

1. **Olfactory receptor cells** are first-order neurons that project to the mitral cells and tufted cells of the olfactory bulb.
2. **Mitral cells** are the principal cells of the olfactory bulb. They are excitatory and glutaminergic. They project through the **olfactory tract** and **lateral olfactory stria** to the primary olfactory cortex and amygdala.
3. **The primary olfactory cortex (Brodmann area 34)** consists of the piriform cortex that overlies the uncus.

B. Lesions of the Olfactory Pathway
result from trauma (e.g., skull fracture) and olfactory groove meningiomas. These lesions cause **ipsilateral anosmia** (loss of olfactory sensation). Lesions that involve the parahippocampal uncus may cause olfactory hallucinations (uncinate fits [seizures] with déjà vu).

C. Foster Kennedy Syndrome
consists of ipsilateral anosmia, ipsilateral optic atrophy, and contralateral papilledema. It is usually caused by an anterior cranial fossa meningioma.

II **The Optic Nerve (CN II)** is a special somatic afferent **(SSA)** nerve that subserves vision and pupillary light reflexes (afferent limb; see Chapter 14). It enters the cranial cavity through the optic canal of the sphenoid bone. It is **not a true peripheral nerve** but is a tract of the diencephalon. A transected optic nerve cannot regenerate. For clinical correlations, see Chapter 14 on Visual System.

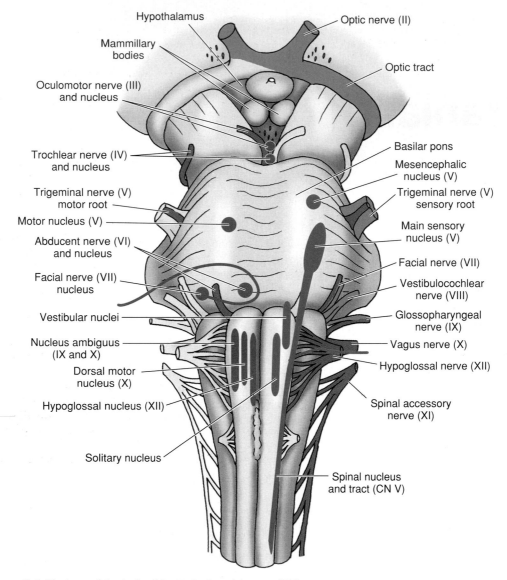

Figure 9-1 The base of the brain with attached cranial nerves (*CN*).

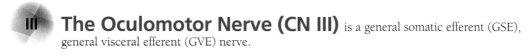

III **The Oculomotor Nerve (CN III)** is a general somatic efferent (GSE), general visceral efferent (GVE) nerve.

A. General Characteristics. The oculomotor nerve **moves** the **eye, constricts** the **pupil, accommodates,** and **converges.** It exits the brain stem from the interpeduncular fossa of the midbrain, passes through the lateral wall of the cavernous sinus, and enters the orbit through the superior orbital fissure.

    1. The **GSE component** arises from the oculomotor nucleus of the rostral midbrain. It innervates four extraocular muscles and the levator palpebrae superioris. (**Remember** the mnemonic **SIN:** **s**uperior muscles are **in**torters of the globe.)

        a. The **medial rectus** adducts the eye. With its opposite partner, it converges the eyes.

        b. The **superior rectus** elevates, intorts, and adducts the eye.

    c. The **inferior rectus** depresses, extorts, and adducts the eye.

    d. The **inferior oblique** elevates, extorts, and abducts the eye.

    e. The **levator palpebrae superioris** elevates the upper eyelid.

2. The **GVE component** consists of preganglionic parasympathetic fibers.

    a. The **accessory oculomotor nucleus (Edinger–Westphal nucleus)** projects preganglionic parasympathetic fibers to the ciliary ganglion of the orbit through CN III.

    b. The **ciliary ganglion** projects postganglionic parasympathetic fibers to the sphincter pupillae (miosis) and the ciliaris (accommodation).

B. Clinical Correlation

1. **Oculomotor paralysis** (palsy) is seen with transtentorial herniation (e.g., tumor, subdural or epidural hematoma).

    a. **Denervation** of the **levator palpebrae superioris** causes **ptosis** (i.e., drooping of the upper eyelid).

    b. **Denervation** of the **extraocular muscles** innervated by CN III causes the affected eye to look "down and out" as a result of the unopposed action of the lateral rectus and superior oblique. The superior oblique and lateral rectus are innervated by CNs IV and VI, respectively. Oculomotor palsy results in **diplopia** (double vision) when the patient looks in the direction of the paretic muscle.

    c. **Interruption of parasympathetic innervation** (internal ophthalmoplegia) results in a **dilated, fixed pupil** and **paralysis of accommodation** (cycloplegia).

2. **Other conditions associated with CN III impairment**

    a. **Transtentorial (uncal) herniation.** Increased supratentorial pressure (e.g., from a tumor) forces the hippocampal uncus through the tentorial notch and compresses or stretches the oculomotor nerve.

      i. **Sphincter pupillae fibers** are affected first, resulting in a **dilated, fixed pupil.**

      ii. **Somatic efferent fibers** are affected later, resulting in **external strabismus** (exotropia).

    b. **Aneurysms** of the carotid and posterior communicating arteries often compress CN III within the cavernous sinus or interpeduncular cistern. They usually affect the peripheral pupilloconstrictor fibers first (e.g., uncal herniation).

    c. **Diabetes mellitus (diabetic oculomotor palsy)** often affects the oculomotor nerve. It damages the central fibers and spares the sphincter pupillae fibers.

 IV **The Trochlear Nerve (CN IV)** is a **GSE** nerve.

A. General Characteristics.
The trochlear nerve is a pure motor nerve that innervates the superior oblique. This muscle depresses, intorts, and abducts the eye (Figure 9-2).

1. It **arises from** the contralateral trochlear nucleus of the caudal midbrain.

2. It **decussates** inferior to the superior medullary velum of the midbrain and exits the brainstem on its posterior surface, caudal to the inferior colliculus.

3. It **encircles the midbrain** within the subarachnoid space, passes through the lateral wall of the cavernous sinus, and enters the orbit through the superior orbital fissure.

B. Clinical Correlation.
Because of its course around the midbrain, the trochlear nerve is particularly vulnerable to head trauma. The trochlear decussation underlies the superior medullary velum. Trauma at this site often results in bilateral fourth-nerve palsies. Pressure against the free border of the tentorium (herniation) may injure the nerve (Figure 9-2). **CN IV paralysis** results in the following conditions:

1. **Extorsion of the eye** and weakness of downward gaze.

2. **Vertical diplopia,** which increases when looking down.

3. **Head tilting** to compensate for extorsion (may be misdiagnosed as idiopathic torticollis).

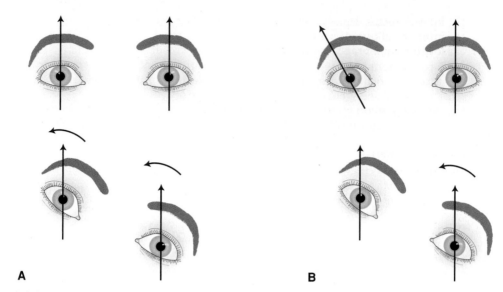

Figure 9-2 Paralysis of the right superior oblique. **A.** A pair of eyes with normal extorsion and intorsion movements. Tilting the chin to the right side results in compensatory intorsion of the left eye and extorsion of the right eye. **B.** Paralysis of the right superior oblique muscle results in extorsion of the right eye, causing diplopia. Tilting the chin to the right side results in compensatory intorsion of the left eye, thus permitting binocular alignment.

 The Trigeminal Nerve (CN V) is a special visceral efferent (SVE) and general somatic afferent (GSA) nerve (Figure 9-3).

A. General Characteristics. The trigeminal nerve is the nerve of pharyngeal (branchial) arch 1 (mandibular). It has three divisions: ophthalmic (CN V_1), maxillary (CN V_2), and mandibular (CN V_3).

1. The **SVE component** arises from the trigeminal motor nucleus that is found in the lateral mid-pontine tegmentum. It **innervates** the **muscles of mastication** (i.e., temporalis, masseter, lateral, and medial pterygoids), the tensors tympani and palati, the mylohyoid, and the anterior belly of the digastric.

2. The **GSA component** provides **sensory innervation** from the face, mucous membranes of the nasal and oral cavities and frontal sinus, hard palate, and deep structures of the head (proprioception from muscles and the temporomandibular joint). It innervates the dura of the anterior and middle cranial fossae (supratentorial dura).

B. Clinical Correlation. Lesions result in the following neurologic deficits:

1. **Loss of general sensation (hemianesthesia)** from the face and mucous membranes of the oral and nasal cavities.

2. **Loss of the corneal reflex** (afferent limb, CN V_1; Figure 9-4).

3. **Flaccid paralysis** of the muscles of mastication.

4. **Deviation of the jaw to the weak side** as a result of the unopposed action of the opposite lateral pterygoid muscle.

5. **Paralysis of the tensor tympani muscle,** which leads to hypoacusis (partial deafness to low-pitched sounds).

6. **Trigeminal neuralgia** (tic douloureux), which is characterized by recurrent paroxysms of sharp, stabbing pain in one or more branches of the nerve.

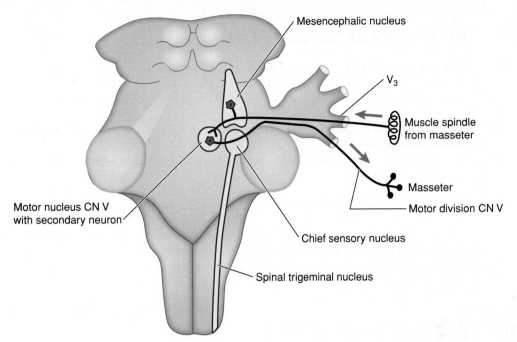

Figure 9-3 Jaw jerk (masseter reflex) pathway showing two neurons. Note that the first-order (sensory) neuron is found in the mesencephalic nucleus of the pons and midbrain, not in the trigeminal ganglion. *CN*, cranial nerve.

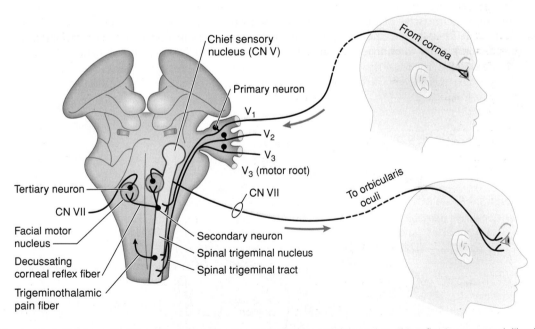

Figure 9-4 The corneal reflex pathway showing the three neurons and decussation. This reflex is consensual, like the pupillary light reflex. Second-order pain neurons are found in the caudal division of the spinal trigeminal nucleus. Second-order corneal reflex neurons are found at more rostral levels. *CN*, cranial nerve.

VI   The Abducent Nerve (CN VI)

A. General Characteristics. The abducent nerve is a pure **GSE nerve** that innervates the lateral rectus, which abducts the eye.

1. It arises from the abducent nucleus that is found in the posteromedial tegmentum of the caudal pons.

2. Exiting intra-axial fibers pass through the corticospinal tract. A **lesion** results in **alternating abducent hemiparesis.**

3. It passes through the pontine cistern and cavernous sinus and enters the orbit through the superior orbital fissure.

B. Clinical Correlation. CN VI Paralysis is the most common isolated palsy that results from the long peripheral course of the nerve. It is seen in patients with meningitis, subarachnoid hemorrhage, late-stage syphilis, and trauma. **Abducent nerve paralysis** results in the **following defects:**

1. **Convergent (medial) strabismus (esotropia)** with inability to abduct the eye.

2. **Horizontal diplopia** with maximum separation of the double images when looking toward the paretic lateral rectus.

VII   The Facial Nerve (CN VII)

A. General Characteristics. The facial nerve is a **GSA, general visceral afferent (GVA), SVA, GVE,** and **SVE** nerve (Figures 9-5 and 9-6). It **mediates facial movements, taste, salivation, lacrimation,** and **general sensation from the external ear.** It is the nerve of the pharyngeal (branchial) arch 2 (hyoid). It includes the facial nerve proper (motor division), which contains the SVE fibers that **innervate the muscles of facial (mimetic) expression.** CN VII includes the intermediate nerve, which contains GSA, SVA, and GVE fibers. All first-order sensory neuronal cell bodies are found in the geniculate ganglion within the temporal bone.

1. **Anatomy.** The facial nerve exits the brain stem in the cerebellopontine angle. It enters the internal auditory meatus and the facial canal. It then exits the facial canal and skull through the stylomastoid foramen.

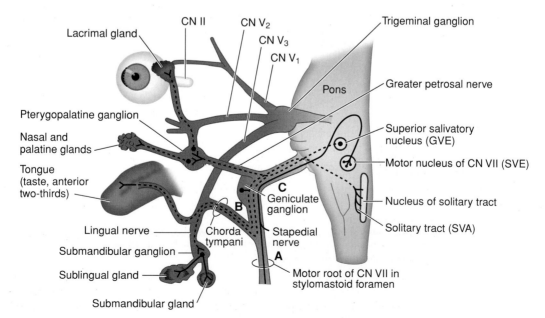

Figure 9-5 The functional components of the facial nerve (cranial nerve [*CN*] VII).

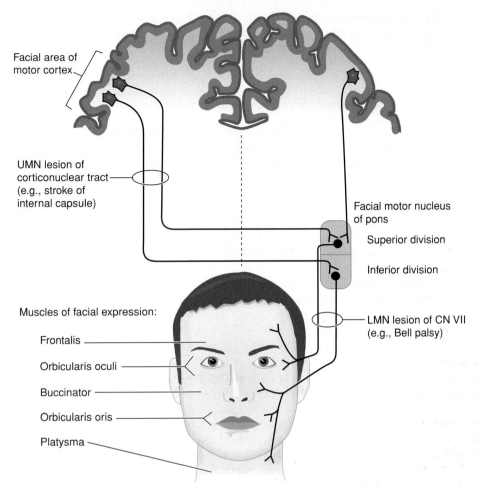

Figure 9-6 Corticonuclear innervation of the facial nerve (cranial nerve [*CN*] VII) nucleus. An upper motor neuron (*UMN*) lesion (e.g., stroke involving the internal capsule) results in contralateral weakness of the lower face, with sparing of the upper face. A lower motor neuron (*LMN*) lesion (e.g., Bell palsy) results in paralysis of the facial muscles in both the upper and lower face. (Redrawn from DeMyer WE. *Technique of the Neurological Examination: A Programmed Text.* 4th ed. New York: McGraw-Hill; 1994:177, with permission.)

2. **The GSA component** has cell bodies located in the geniculate ganglion. It innervates the posterior surface of the external ear through the posterior auricular branch of CN VII. It projects centrally to the spinal tract and nucleus of trigeminal nerve.

3. **The GVA component** has no clinical significance. The cell bodies are located in the geniculate ganglion. Fibers innervate the soft palate and the adjacent pharyngeal wall.

4. **The SVA component (taste)** has cell bodies located in the geniculate ganglion. It projects centrally to the solitary tract and nucleus. It innervates the taste buds from the anterior two-thirds of the tongue through:

   a. The **intermediate nerve.**

   b. The **chorda tympani,** which is located in the tympanic cavity medial to the tympanic membrane and malleus. It contains the SVA and GVE (parasympathetic) fibers.

   c. The **lingual nerve** (a branch of CN V$_3$).

   d. The **central gustatory pathway** (see Figure 9-5). Taste fibers from CNs VII, IX, and X project through the solitary tract to the solitary nucleus. The solitary nucleus projects through the central tegmental tract to the ventral posteromedial nucleus (VPM) of the thalamus. The VPM projects to the gustatory cortex of the parietal lobe (parietal operculum).

5. **The GVE component** is a parasympathetic component that innervates the lacrimal, submandibular, and sublingual glands. It contains preganglionic parasympathetic neurons that are located in the superior salivatory nucleus of the caudal pons.
   a. **Lacrimal pathway** (see Figure 9-5). The superior salivatory nucleus projects through the intermediate and greater petrosal nerves to the pterygopalatine ganglion. Postganglionic neurons from the pterygopalatine ganglion project through the inferior orbital fissure and travel via the zygomatic nerve (a branch of V$_2$) and lacrimal nerve (a branch of V$_1$) to innervate the lacrimal gland.
   b. **Submandibular pathway** (see Figure 9-5). The superior salivatory nucleus projects through the intermediate nerve and chorda tympani to the submandibular ganglion. Postganglionic neurons from the submandibular ganglion project to and innervate the submandibular and sublingual glands.
6. **The SVE component** arises from the facial motor nucleus, loops around the abducent nucleus of the caudal pons, and exits the brain stem in the cerebellopontine angle. It enters the internal auditory meatus, traverses the facial canal, sends a branch to the stapedius in the middle ear, and exits the skull through the stylomastoid foramen. It innervates the muscles of facial expression, the stylohyoid, the posterior belly of the digastric, and the stapedius.

B. Clinical Correlation. Lesions cause the following conditions:
1. **Flaccid paralysis** of the **muscles of facial expression** (upper and lower face).
2. **Loss of the corneal (blink) reflex** (efferent limb), which may lead to corneal ulceration (keratitis paralytica).
3. **Loss of taste** (ageusia) from the anterior two-thirds of the tongue, which may result from damage to the chorda tympani.
4. **Hyperacusis** (increased acuity to sounds) as a result of stapedius paralysis.
5. **Bell palsy** (peripheral facial paralysis), which is caused by a lower motor neuron lesion resulting from trauma or infection. This palsy involves the upper and lower face.
6. **Crocodile tears syndrome** (lacrimation during eating), which is a result of aberrant regeneration of GVE fibers after trauma. Regenerating preganglionic salivary fibers are misdirected to the pterygopalatine ganglion which projects to the lacrimal gland.
7. **Supranuclear (central) facial palsy,** which is caused by an upper motor neuron lesion and results in contralateral weakness of the lower face, with sparing of the upper face (see Figure 9-6).
8. **Bilateral facial nerve palsies,** which occur in Guillain–Barré syndrome.
9. **Möbius syndrome,** which consists of congenital facial diplegia (CN VII) and convergent strabismus (CN VI).

VIII The Vestibulocochlear Nerve (CN VIII) is an SSA nerve. It has two
functional divisions: the vestibular nerve, which **maintains equilibrium and balance,** and the cochlear nerve, which **mediates hearing.** It exits the brain stem at the cerebellopontine angle and enters the internal auditory meatus. It is confined to the temporal bone.

A. Vestibular Nerve (see Figure 13-1)
1. **General characteristics**
   a. It is associated functionally with the cerebellum (flocculonodular lobe) and ocular motor nuclei.
   b. It regulates compensatory eye movements.
   c. Its first-order neuronal cell bodies are located in the vestibular ganglion in the fundus of the internal auditory meatus.
   d. It projects its peripheral processes to the hair cells of the cristae of the semicircular ducts and the hair cells of the utricle and saccule.
   e. It projects its central processes to the four vestibular nuclei of the brain stem and the flocculonodular lobe of the cerebellum.
   f. It conducts efferent fibers to the hair cells from the brain stem.
2. **Clinical correlation.** Lesions result in **disequilibrium, vertigo,** and **nystagmus.**

B. Cochlear Nerve (see Figure 12-1)

1. **General characteristics**
   a. Its first-order neuronal cell bodies are located in the spiral (cochlear) ganglion of the modiolus of the cochlea, within the temporal bone.
   b. It projects its peripheral processes to the hair cells of the organ of Corti.
   c. It projects its central processes to the dorsal and ventral cochlear nuclei of the brain stem.
   d. It conducts efferent fibers to the hair cells from the brain stem.

2. **Clinical correlation.** Destructive lesions cause **hearing loss** (sensorineural deafness). Irritative lesions can cause **tinnitus** (ear ringing). An **acoustic neuroma** (schwannoma) is a Schwann cell tumor of the cochlear nerve that causes deafness.

IX The Glossopharyngeal Nerve (CN IX) is a GSA, GVA, SVA, SVE, and **GVE** nerve.

A. General Characteristics. The glossopharyngeal nerve is primarily a sensory nerve. Along with CNs VII and X, it **mediates taste, salivation,** and **swallowing. It mediates input** from the **carotid sinus,** which contains baroreceptors that monitor arterial blood pressure. It also **mediates input** from the **carotid body,** which contains chemoreceptors that monitor the CO_2 and O_2 concentration of the blood.

1. **Anatomy.** CN IX is the nerve of pharyngeal (branchial) arch 3. It exits the brain stem (medulla) from the postolivary sulcus with CNs X and XI. It exits the skull through the jugular foramen with CNs X and XI.

2. **The GSA component** innervates part of the external ear and the external auditory meatus through the auricular branch of the vagus nerve. It has cell bodies in the superior ganglion. It projects its central processes to the spinal tract and nucleus of trigeminal nerve.

3. **The GVA component** innervates structures that are derived from the endoderm (e.g., pharynx). It **innervates** the **mucous membranes** of the posterior one-third of the tongue, tonsil, upper pharynx, tympanic cavity, and auditory tube. It also **innervates** the **carotid sinus** (baroreceptors) and **carotid body** (chemoreceptors) through the sinus nerve. It has cell bodies in the inferior (petrosal) ganglion. It is the afferent limb of the gag reflex and the carotid sinus reflex.

4. **The SVA component** innervates the taste buds of the posterior one-third of the tongue. It has cell bodies in the inferior (petrosal) ganglion. It projects its central processes to the solitary tract and nucleus.

5. **The SVE component** innervates only the stylopharyngeus muscle. It arises from the nucleus ambiguus of the lateral medulla.

6. **The GVE component** is a parasympathetic component that innervates the parotid gland. Preganglionic parasympathetic neurons are located in the inferior salivatory nucleus of the medulla. They project through the tympanic and lesser petrosal nerves to the otic ganglion. Postganglionic fibers from the otic ganglion project to the parotid gland through the auriculotemporal nerve (CN V_3).

B. Clinical Correlation. Lesions cause the following conditions:

1. **Loss of the gag (pharyngeal) reflex** (interruption of the afferent limb).
2. **Hypersensitive carotid sinus reflex** (syncope).
3. **Loss of general sensation** in the **pharynx, tonsils, fauces,** and **back of the tongue.**
4. **Loss of taste** from the posterior one-third of the tongue.
5. **Glossopharyngeal neuralgia,** which is characterized by severe stabbing pain in the root of the tongue.

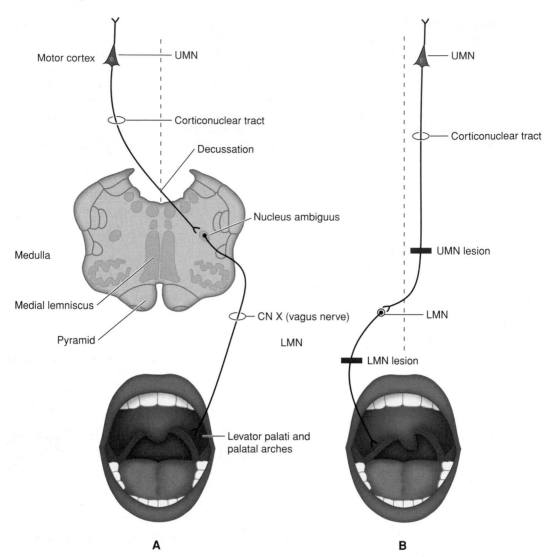

Figure 9-7 Innervation of the palatal arches and uvula. Sensory innervation is mediated by the glossopharyngeal nerve (cranial nerve [*CN*] IX). Motor innervation of the palatal arches and uvula is mediated by the vagus nerve (CN X). **A.** A normal palate and uvula in a person who is saying "Ah." **B.** A patient with an upper motor neuron (*UMN*) lesion (left) and a lower motor neuron (*LMN*) lesion (right). When this patient says "Ah," the palatal arches sag. The uvula deviates toward the intact (left) side.

 X   **The Vagal Nerve (CN X)** is a **GSA, GVA, SVA, SVE,** and **GVE** nerve (see Figure 9-7).

A. General Characteristics. The vagal nerve **mediates phonation, swallowing** (with CNs IX, XI, and XII), elevation of the palate, taste, and cutaneous sensation from the ear. **It innervates the viscera** of the **neck, thorax,** and **abdomen.**

    1. Anatomy. The vagal nerve is the nerve of pharyngeal (branchial) arches 4 and 6. Pharyngeal arch 5 is either absent or rudimentary. It exits the brain stem (medulla) from the postolivary sulcus. It exits the skull through the jugular foramen with CNs IX and XI.

2. **The GSA component** innervates the infratentorial dura, external ear, external auditory meatus, and external surface of the tympanic membrane. It has cell bodies in the superior (jugular) ganglion, and it projects its central processes to the spinal tract and nucleus of trigeminal nerve.

3. **The GVA component** innervates the mucous membranes of the pharynx, larynx, esophagus, trachea, and thoracic and abdominal viscera (to the midtransverse colon). It has cell bodies in the inferior (nodose) ganglion. It projects its central processes to the solitary tract and nucleus.

4. **The SVA component** innervates the taste buds in the epiglottic region. It has cell bodies in the inferior (nodose) ganglion. It projects its central processes to the solitary tract and nucleus.

5. **The SVE component** innervates the pharyngeal (brachial) arch muscles of the larynx and pharynx, the striated muscle of the upper esophagus, musculus uvulae, levator palati, and palatoglossus. It arises from the nucleus ambiguus in the lateral medulla. The SVE component provides the efferent limb of the gag reflex.

6. **The GVE component** innervates the viscera of the neck and the thoracic (heart) and abdominal cavities as far as the midtransverse colon. Preganglionic parasympathetic neurons that are located in the dorsal motor nucleus of the medulla project to the terminal (intramural) ganglia of the visceral organs.

B. Clinical Correlation. Lesions and **reflexes** cause the following conditions:

1. **Ipsilateral paralysis** of the soft palate, pharynx, and larynx that leads to dysphonia (hoarseness), dyspnea, dysarthria, and dysphagia.

2. **Loss of the gag (palatal) reflex** (efferent limb).

3. **Anesthesia of the pharynx and larynx** that leads to unilateral loss of the cough reflex.

4. **Aortic aneurysms and tumors** of the neck and thorax that frequently compress the vagal nerve and can lead to cough, dyspnea, dysphagia, hoarseness, and chest/back pain.

5. **Complete laryngeal paralysis,** which can be rapidly fatal if it is bilateral (asphyxia).

6. **Parasympathetic (vegetative) disturbances,** including bradycardia (irritative lesion), tachycardia (destructive lesion), and dilation of the stomach.

7. The **oculocardiac reflex,** in which pressure on the eye slows the heart rate (afferent limb of CN V_1 and efferent limb of CN X).

8. The **carotid sinus reflex,** in which pressure on the carotid sinus slows the heart rate (bradycardia; efferent limb of CN X).

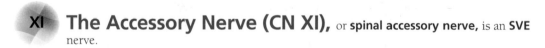

XI The Accessory Nerve (CN XI), or **spinal accessory nerve,** is an **SVE** nerve.

A. General Characteristics. The accessory nerve **mediates head and shoulder movement.** It arises from the anterior horn of cervical spinal cord segments C1 through C6. The spinal roots exit the spinal cord laterally between the anterior and posterior spinal roots, ascend through the foramen magnum, and exit the skull through the jugular foramen. It **innervates** the **sternocleidomastoid** and the **trapezius.**

B. Clinical Correlation. Lesions cause the following conditions:

1. **Paralysis of the sternocleidomastoid** results in difficulty in turning the head to the contralateral side.

2. **Paralysis of the trapezius muscle** results in shoulder droop and inability to shrug the shoulder.

XII The Hypoglossal Nerve (CN XII) is a **GSE** nerve.

A. General Characteristics. The hypoglossal nerve **mediates tongue movement.** It arises from the hypoglossal motor nucleus of the medulla and exits the medulla in the preolivary sulcus. It exits the skull through the hypoglossal canal, and it **innervates** the **intrinsic and extrinsic muscles**

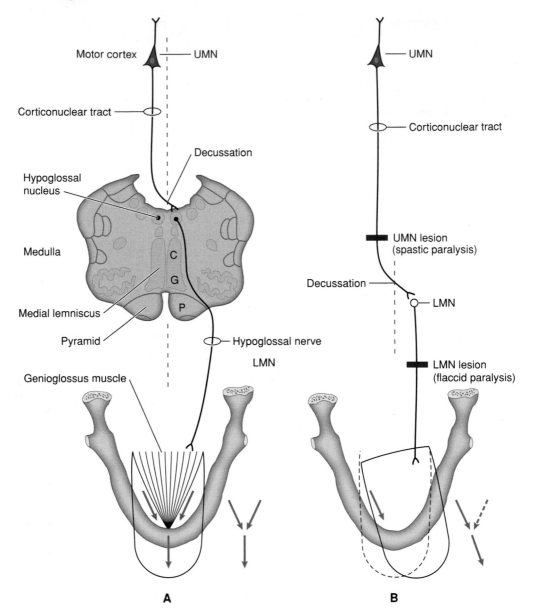

Figure 9-8 Motor innervation of the tongue. Corticonuclear fibers project predominantly to the contralateral hypo-glossal motor nucleus. An upper motor neuron (*UMN*) lesion causes deviation of the protruded tongue to the weak (contralateral) side. A lower motor neuron (*LMN*) lesion causes deviation of the protruded tongue to the weak (ipsilateral) side. **A.** Normal tongue. **B.** Tongue with UMN and LMN lesions.

of the **tongue.** Extrinsic muscles are the genioglossus, styloglossus, and hyoglossus (palatoglossus is considered a muscle of the soft palate and is innervated by CN X).

B. Clinical Correlation

1. **Transection** results in hemiparalysis of the tongue.
2. **Protrusion** causes the tongue to point toward the lesioned (weak) side because of the unopposed action of the opposite genioglossus muscle (Figure 9-8).

CHAPTER 10

Trigeminal System

Objectives

1. List the central and peripheral components of the trigeminal system, including the location and function of the appropriate nuclei.
2. Describe the divisions of the trigeminal nerve, including the fiber types in each division and their targets.
3. Diagram the ascending trigeminothalamic pathways, including the constituent primary, secondary, and tertiary neurons. List all cranial nerves that utilize these pathways.

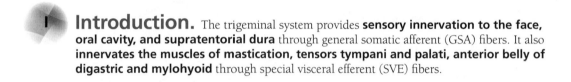

I **Introduction.** The trigeminal system provides **sensory innervation to the face, oral cavity, and supratentorial dura** through general somatic afferent (GSA) fibers. It also **innervates the muscles of mastication, tensors tympani and palati, anterior belly of digastric and mylohyoid** through special visceral efferent (SVE) fibers.

II **The Trigeminal Ganglion** (semilunar or gasserian) contains pseudounipolar ganglion cells. It has three divisions:

A. The **ophthalmic nerve (cranial nerve CN V₁)** lies in the lateral wall of the cavernous sinus. It enters the orbit through the superior orbital fissure and innervates the forehead, dorsum of the nose, upper eyelid, orbit (cornea and conjunctiva), and cranial dura. The ophthalmic nerve mediates the afferent limb of the corneal reflex.

B. The **maxillary nerve (CN V₂)** lies in the lateral wall of the cavernous sinus and innervates the upper lip and cheek, lower eyelid, anterior portion of the temple, oral mucosa of the upper mouth, nose, pharynx, gums, teeth and palate of the upper jaw, and cranial dura. It exits the skull through the foramen rotundum.

C. The **mandibular nerve (CN V₃)** exits the skull through the foramen ovale. Its **sensory (GSA) component** innervates the lower lip and chin, posterior portion of the temple, external auditory meatus, and tympanic membrane, external ear, teeth of the lower jaw, oral mucosa of the cheeks and floor of the mouth, anterior two-thirds of the tongue, temporomandibular joint, and cranial dura. The **motor (SVE) component** of CN V accompanies the mandibular nerve (CN V₃) through the foramen ovale. It innervates the muscles of mastication, mylohyoid, anterior belly of the digastric, and tensors tympani and palati (Figure 10-1).

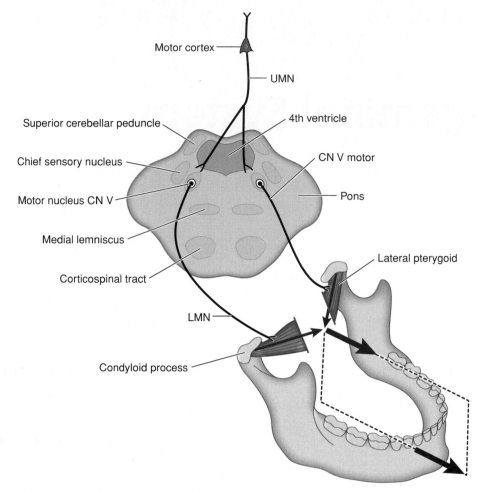

Figure 10-1 Function and innervation of the lateral pterygoid muscles (LPMs). The LPM receives its innervation from the trigeminal motor nucleus found in the rostral pons. Bilateral innervation of the LPMs results in protrusion of the mandible in the midline. The LPMs also depress the mandible. Denervation of one LPM results in deviation of the mandible to the ipsilateral or weak side. The trigeminal motor nucleus receives bilateral corticonuclear input. *CN,* cranial nerve; *LMN,* lower motor neuron; *UMN,* upper motor neuron.

 III   **Trigeminothalamic Pathways** (Figure 10-2)

A. The **anterior trigeminothalamic tract** mediates pain and temperature sensation from the face and oral cavity.

    1. First-order neurons are located in the trigeminal (gasserian) ganglion. They give rise to axons that descend in the spinal tract of trigeminal nerve and synapse with second-order neurons in the spinal nucleus of trigeminal nerve.

    2. Second-order neurons are located in the spinal trigeminal nucleus. They give rise to decussating axons that terminate in the contralateral ventral posteromedial (VPM) nucleus of the thalamus.

    3. Third-order neurons are located in the VPM nucleus of the thalamus. They project through the posterior limb of the internal capsule to the face area of the somatosensory cortex (Brodmann areas 3, 1, and 2).

B. The **posterior trigeminothalamic tract** mediates tactile discrimination and pressure sensation from the face and oral cavity. It receives input from Meissner and Pacinian corpuscles.

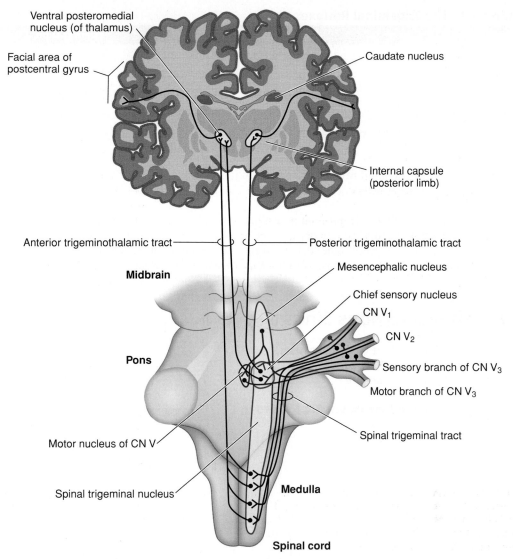

Figure 10-2 The anterior (pain and temperature) and posterior (discriminative touch) trigeminothalamic pathways. *CN*, cranial nerve.

1. **First-order neurons** are located in the trigeminal (gasserian) ganglion. They synapse in the principal sensory nucleus of CN V.
2. **Second-order neurons** are located in the principal sensory nucleus of CN V. They project to the ipsilateral VPM nucleus of the thalamus.
3. **Third-order neurons** are located in the VPM nucleus of the thalamus. They project through the posterior limb of the internal capsule to the face area of the somatosensory cortex (Brodmann areas 3, 1, and 2).

IV Trigeminal Reflexes

A. Introduction (Table 10-1)
1. The **corneal reflex** is a consensual and disynaptic reflex.
2. The **jaw jerk reflex** is a monosynaptic myotactic reflex (Figure 10-3).

Table 10-1: The Trigeminal Reflexes

Reflex	Afferent Limb	Efferent Limb
Corneal reflex	Ophthalmic nerve (CN V₁)	Facial nerve (CN VII)
Jaw jerk	Mandibular nerve (CN V₃)[a]	Mandibular nerve (CN V₃)
Tearing (lacrimal) reflex	Ophthalmic nerve (CN V₁)	Facial nerve (CN VII)
Oculocardiac reflex	Ophthalmic nerve (CN V₁)	Vagal nerve (CN X)

[a]The cell bodies are found in the mesencephalic nucleus of CN V.
CN, cranial nerve.

3. The **tearing (lacrimal) reflex** occurs as a result of corneal or conjunctival irritation.
4. The **oculocardiac reflex** occurs when pressure on the globe results in **bradycardia.**

B. Clinical Correlation. Trigeminal neuralgia (tic douloureux) is characterized by recurrent paroxysms of sharp, stabbing pain in one or more branches of the trigeminal nerve on one side of the face. It usually occurs in people older than 50 years, and it is more common in women than in men. **Carbamazepine** is the drug of choice for idiopathic trigeminal neuralgia.

 V **The Cavernous Sinus** (Figure 10-4) contains the following structures:

A. Internal Carotid Artery (Siphon)

B. CNs III, IV, V₁, V₂, and VI

C. Postganglionic Sympathetic Fibers en route to the orbit

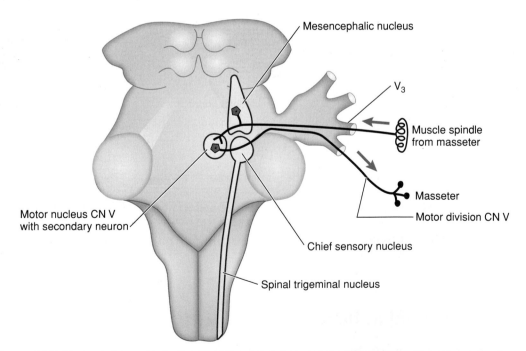

Figure 10-3 The jaw jerk (masseter) reflex. The afferent limb is V₃, and the efferent limb is the motor root that accompanies V₃. First-order sensory neurons are located in the mesencephalic nucleus. The jaw jerk reflex, like all muscle stretch reflexes, is a monosynaptic myotactic reflex. Hyperreflexia indicates an upper motor neuron lesion. *CN*, cranial nerve.

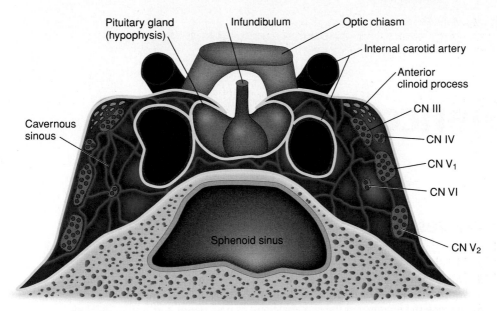

Figure 10-4 The contents of the cavernous sinus. The lateral wall of the cavernous sinus contains the ophthalmic cranial nerve (CN V$_1$) and maxillary (CN V$_2$) divisions of the trigeminal nerve (CN V) and the trochlear (CN IV) and oculomotor (CN III) nerves. The siphon of the internal carotid artery and the abducent nerve (CN VI), along with postganglionic sympathetic fibers, lie within the cavernous sinus. (Modified from Fix JD. High-Yield Neuroanatomy. 3rd ed. Philadelphia, PA: Lippincott Williams & Wilkins; 2005:81, and Gould DJ, Fix JD. BRS Neuroanatomy 5th ed. Philadelphia, PA: 2014, Lippincott, Williams & Wilkins, a Wolters Kluwer business.)

CASE 10-1

A 50-year-old woman complains of sudden onset of pain over the left side of her lower face, with the attacks consisting of brief shocks of pain that last only a few seconds at a time. Between episodes, she has no pain. Usually, the attacks are triggered by brushing her teeth, and they extend from her ear to her chin. What is the most likely diagnosis?

Relevant Physical Exam Findings

● Neurologic exam was normal to motor, sensory, and reflex testing. Magnetic resonance imaging findings were normal as well.

Diagnosis

● Trigeminal neuralgia (tic douloureux)

CHAPTER 11

Diencephalon

Objectives

1. List the thalamic nuclei and attribute at least one main functional association to each.
2. Describe the internal capsule's parts and what fibers travel within each.
3. Identify the internal capsule and surrounding structures on an image or diagram.
4. List the hypothalamic nuclei and attribute at least one main functional association to each.
5. Describe the anatomy of the hypothalamus, its boundaries and various divisions.
6. Describe the "systems" associated with hypothalamic regions, for example, the heat regulation or satiety centers.

I **Introduction.** The diencephalon is divided into four parts: the subthalamus, epithalamus, dorsal thalamus (i.e., the thalamus), and the hypothalamus. The **epithalamus** includes the **pineal gland,** which in humans has a role in circadian rhythms and reproductive cycles and the **habenula,** which has connections between the basal nuclei, limbic system, and brainstem reticular formation. The **subthalamus** is region that is essentially a continuation of the midbrain tegmentum, the main component is the **subthalamic nucleus,** which functions as part of the basal nuclei.

II **The thalamus** is the largest division of the diencephalon. It plays an important role in the integration of the sensory and motor systems.

Major Thalamic Nuclei and Their Connections (Figure 11-1)

A. The **anterior nucleus** receives hypothalamic input from the mammillary nucleus through the mammillothalamic tract. It projects to the cingulate gyrus and is part of the Papez circuit of emotion of the limbic system.

B. The **mediodorsal (dorsomedial) nucleus** is reciprocally connected to the prefrontal cortex. It has abundant connections with the intralaminar nuclei. It receives input from the amygdala, substantia nigra, and temporal neocortex. When it is destroyed, **memory loss** occurs (Wernicke–Korsakoff syndrome). The mediodorsal nucleus plays a role in the expression of affect, emotion, and behavior (limbic function).

C. The **centromedian nucleus** is the largest intralaminar nucleus. It is reciprocally connected to the motor cortex (Brodmann area 4). The centromedian nucleus receives input from the globus pallidus. It projects to the striatum (caudate nucleus and putamen) and projects diffusely to the entire neocortex.

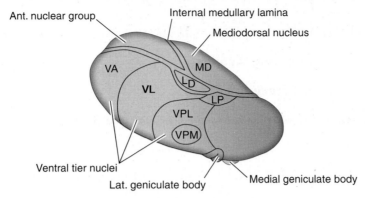

Figure 11-1 Major thalamic nuclei and their connections. **A.** Dorsolateral aspect and major nuclei. *LD,* lateral dorsal nucleus; *LP,* lateral posterior nucleus; *MD,* medial dorsal nucleus; *VA,* ventral anterior nucleus; *VL,* ventral lateral nucleus; *VPL,* ventral posterior lateral nucleus; *VPM,* ventral posterior medial nucleus.

D. The **pulvinar** is the largest thalamic nucleus. It has reciprocal connections with the association cortex of the occipital, parietal, and posterior temporal lobes. It receives input from the lateral and medial geniculate bodies and the superior colliculus. It plays a role in the **integration of visual, auditory, and somesthetic input.** Destruction of the pulvinar may result in sensory dysphasia.

E. Ventral Tier Nuclei

1. The **ventral anterior nucleus** receives input from the globus pallidus and substantia nigra. It projects diffusely to the prefrontal cortex, orbital cortex, and premotor cortex (Brodmann area 6).
2. The **ventral lateral nucleus** receives input from the cerebellum (dentate nucleus), globus pallidus, and substantia nigra. It projects to the motor cortex (Brodmann area 4) and the supplementary motor cortex (Brodmann area 6).
3. The **ventral posterior nucleus** is the nucleus of termination of general somatic afferent (touch, pain, and temperature) and special visceral afferent (taste) fibers. It has two subnuclei:
   a. **Ventral posterolateral nucleus** receives the spinothalamic tracts and the medial lemniscus. It projects to the somesthetic (sensory) cortex (Brodmann areas 3, 1, and 2);
   b. **Ventral posteromedial (VPM) nucleus** receives the trigeminothalamic tracts and projects to the somesthetic (sensory) cortex (Brodmann areas 3, 1, and 2). The gustatory (taste) pathway originates in the solitary nucleus and projects via the central tegmental tract to the VPM and thence to the gustatory cortex of the postcentral gyrus, of the frontal operculum, and of the insular cortex. The taste pathway is ipsilateral.
4. The **lateral geniculate body** is a visual relay nucleus. It receives retinal input through the optic tract and projects to the primary visual cortex (Brodmann area 17).
5. The **medial geniculate body** is an auditory relay nucleus. It receives auditory input through the brachium of the inferior colliculus and projects to the primary auditory cortex (Brodmann areas 41 and 42).

F. The **reticular nucleus of the thalamus** surrounds the thalamus as a thin layer of γ-aminobutyric acid (GABA)-ergic neurons. It lies between the external medullary lamina and the internal capsule. It receives excitatory collateral input from corticothalamic and thalamocortical fibers. It projects inhibitory fibers to thalamic nuclei, from which it receives input.

III   Blood Supply. The thalamus is irrigated by the following three arteries (see Figure 4-1):

A. Posterior Communicating Artery

B. Posterior Cerebral Artery

C. Anterior Choroidal Artery (Lateral Geniculate Body)

IV   The Internal Capsule (Figure 11-2) is a layer of white matter (myelinated axons) that separates the caudate nucleus and the thalamus medially from the lentiform nucleus laterally. It can be divided into five parts, the:

1. **Anterior limb** is located between the caudate nucleus and the lentiform nucleus (globus pallidus and putamen). It contains fibers that interconnect the anterior nucleus and the cingulate gyrus, as well as fibers connecting the dorsomedial nucleus with the prefrontal cortex. Finally, it contains frontopontine fibers.
2. **Genu** is located near the interventricular foramen and contains corticonuclear fibers.
3. **Posterior limb** is located between the thalamus and the lentiform nucleus. It contains fibers that connect the VA and VL nuclei with motor cortex, as well as fibers connecting the VP nuclei to somatosensory cortex. Descending fibers include corticospinal (pyramid) and corticonuclear fibers.
4. **Retrolenticular part** is composed of fibers passing posteriorly to the lentiform nucleus. This includes the **optic radiations** and fibers that interconnect the pulvinar nucleus with parietal and occipital association cortices.

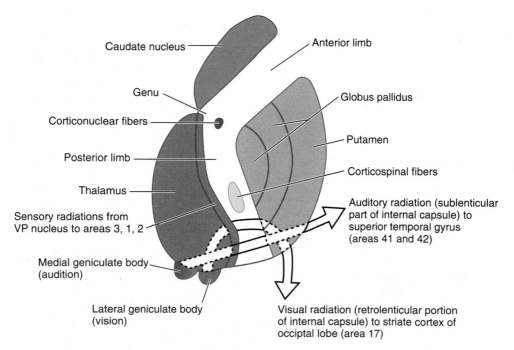

Figure 11-2 Horizontal section of the right internal capsule showing the major fiber projections. Clinically important tracts lie in the genu and posterior limb. Lesions of the internal capsule cause contralateral hemiparesis and contralateral hemianopia. *VP,* ventral posterior.

5. **Sublenticular part** is located inferior to the lentiform nucleus. Sublenticular fibers are composed of the remaining optic radiations, auditory radiations, and interconnections between the temporal association cortices and the pulvinar.

D. Blood Supply to the Internal Capsule

1. The **anterior limb** is irrigated by the medial striate branches of the anterior cerebral artery and the lateral striate (lenticulostriate) branches of the middle cerebral artery.
2. The **genu** is perfused either by direct branches from the internal carotid artery or by pallidal branches of the anterior choroidal artery.
3. The **posterior limb** is supplied by branches of the anterior choroidal artery and lenticulostriate branches of the middle cerebral arteries.
4. The anterior choroidal supplies most of the blood to the retro- and sublenticular parts of the internal capsule.

 The hypothalamus, the inferiormost division of the diencephalon, subserves three systems: the autonomic nervous system, the endocrine system, and the limbic system. The hypothalamus helps to maintain homeostasis. It is bilateral structure, with the inferior recess of the third ventricle intervening between its left and right sides.

A. Major Hypothalamic Nuclei and Their Functions

1. The **medial preoptic nucleus** (Figure 11-3) regulates the release of gonadotropic hormones from the adenohypophysis. It contains the sexually dimorphic nucleus, the development of which depends on testosterone levels.
2. The **suprachiasmatic nucleus** receives direct input from the retina. It plays a role in the regulation of circadian rhythms.
3. The **anterior nucleus** plays a role in temperature regulation. It stimulates the parasympathetic nervous system. Destruction results in hyperthermia.

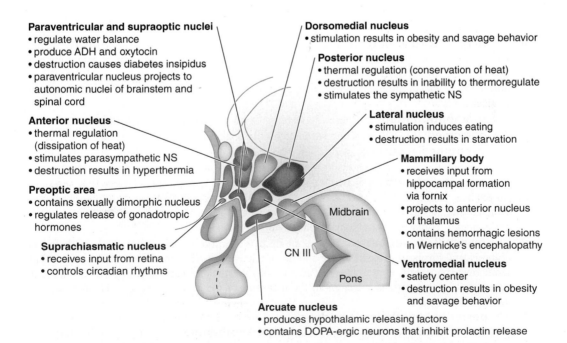

Figure 11-3 Major hypothalamic nuclei and their functions. *ADH,* antidiuretic hormone; *CN,* cranial nerve; *DOPA,* dopamine; *NS,* nervous system.

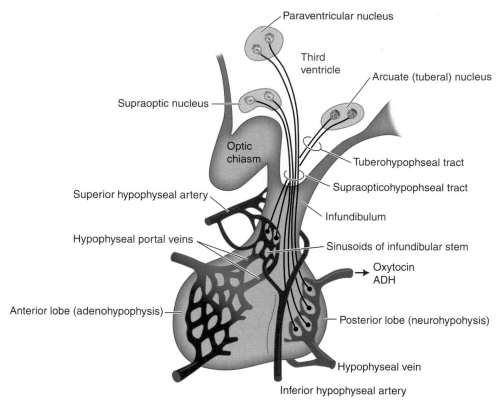

Figure 11-4 The hypophyseal portal system. The paraventricular and supraoptic nuclei produce antidiuretic hormone (*ADH*) and oxytocin and transport them through the supraopticohypophysial tract to the capillary bed of the neurohypophysis. The arcuate nucleus of the infundibulum transports hypothalamic-stimulating hormones through the tuberohypophysial tract to the sinusoids of the infundibular stem. These sinusoids then drain into the secondary capillary plexus in the adenohypophysis.

4. The **paraventricular nucleus** (Figure 11-4) synthesizes antidiuretic hormone (ADH), oxytocin, and corticotropin-releasing hormone. It gives rise to the supraopticohypophyseal tract, which projects to the neurohypophysis. It regulates water balance (conservation) and projects directly to the autonomic nuclei of the brain stem and all levels of the spinal cord. Destruction results in diabetes insipidus.

5. The **supraoptic nucleus** synthesizes ADH and oxytocin (similar to the paraventricular nucleus).

6. The **dorsomedial nucleus,** when stimulated in animals, results in savage behavior.

7. The **ventromedial nucleus** is considered a satiety center. When stimulated, it inhibits the urge to eat. Bilateral destruction results in hyperphagia, obesity, and savage behavior.

8. The **arcuate (infundibular) nucleus** contains neurons that produce factors that stimulate or inhibit the action of the hypothalamus. This nucleus gives rise to the tuberohypophysial tract, which terminates in the hypophyseal portal system (see Figure 11-4) of the infundibulum (medium eminence). It contains neurons that produce dopamine.

9. The **mammillary nucleus** receives input from the hippocampal formation through the postcommissural fornix. It projects to the anterior nucleus of the thalamus through the mammillothalamic tract (part of the Papez circuit). Patients with Wernicke encephalopathy, which is a thiamine (vitamin B_1) deficiency, have lesions in the mammillary nucleus. Lesions are also associated with alcoholism.

10. The **posterior hypothalamic nucleus** plays a role in thermal regulation (i.e., conservation and increased production of heat). Lesions result in **poikilothermia** (i.e., inability to thermoregulate).

11. The **lateral hypothalamic nucleus** induces eating when stimulated. **Lesions** cause **anorexia and starvation.**

B. Major Fiber Systems of the Hypothalamus

1. The **fornix** is the largest projection to the hypothalamus. It projects from the hippocampal formation to the mammillary nucleus, anterior nucleus of the thalamus, and septal area. The fornix then projects from the septal area to the hippocampal formation.

2. The **medial forebrain bundle** traverses the entire lateral hypothalamic area. It interconnects the orbitofrontal cortex, septal area, hypothalamus, and midbrain.

3. The **mammillothalamic tract** projects from the mammillary nuclei to the anterior nucleus of the thalamus (part of the Papez circuit).

4. The **stria terminalis** is the major pathway from the amygdala. It interconnects the septal area, hypothalamus, and amygdala.

5. The **supraopticohypophysial tract** conducts fibers from the supraoptic and paraventricular nuclei to the neurohypophysis, which is the release site for ADH and oxytocin.

6. The **tuberohypophysial (tuberoinfundibular) tract** conducts fibers from the arcuate nucleus to the hypophyseal portal system (see Figure 11-4).

7. The **hypothalamospinal tract** contains direct descending autonomic fibers. These fibers influence the preganglionic sympathetic neurons of the intermediolateral cell column and preganglionic neurons of the sacral parasympathetic nucleus. Interruption above the first thoracic segment (T-1) causes Horner syndrome.

C. Hypothalamic Functional Regions

1. **Autonomic function**
   a. The **anterior hypothalamus** has an excitatory effect on the parasympathetic nervous system. Lesion results in unopposed sympathetic activation.
   b. The **posterior hypothalamus** has an excitatory effect on the sympathetic nervous system. Lesion results in unopposed parasympathetic activation.

2. **Temperature regulation**
   a. The **anterior hypothalamus** regulates and maintains body temperature. Destruction causes hyperthermia.
   b. The **posterior hypothalamus** helps to produce and conserve heat. Destruction causes hypothermia.

3. **Water balance regulation.** The **paraventricular nucleus** synthesizes ADH, which controls water excretion by the kidneys.

4. **Food intake regulation.** Two hypothalamic nuclei play a role in the control of appetite.
   a. When stimulated, the **ventromedial nucleus** inhibits the urge to eat. Bilateral destruction results in hyperphagia, obesity, and savage behavior.
   b. When stimulated, the **lateral hypothalamic nucleus** induces the urge to eat. Destruction causes starvation and emaciation.

D. Hypothalamic Clinical Correlations

1. **Diabetes insipidus,** characterized by polyuria and polydipsia, results from lesions of the ADH pathways to the posterior lobe of the pituitary gland.

2. The **syndrome of inappropriate ADH secretion** may be caused by lung tumors or drug therapy (e.g., carbamazepine, chlorpromazine) and results in hyponatremia.

3. **Craniopharyngioma** is a congenital tumor that originates from remnants of Rathke pouch (see Chapter 2). The tumor is usually calcified. It is the most common supratentorial tumor in children and the most common cause of hypopituitarism in children.
   a. **Pressure on the optic chiasm** results in bitemporal hemianopia.
   b. **Pressure on the hypothalamus** causes hypothalamic syndrome (i.e., adiposity, diabetes insipidus, disturbance of temperature regulation, and somnolence).

E. Pituitary Adenomas account for 15% of clinical symptomatic intracranial tumors. They are rarely seen in children. When pituitary adenomas are endocrine-active, they cause endocrine abnormalities (e.g., amenorrhea and galactorrhea from a prolactin-secreting adenoma, the most common type).

1. **Pressure on the optic chiasm** results in bitemporal hemianopia.
2. **Pressure on the hypothalamus** may cause hypothalamic syndrome (Figure 11-5).

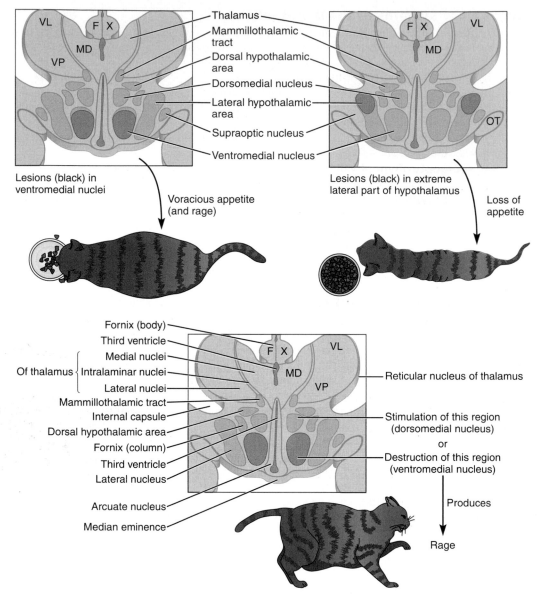

Figure 11-5 Coronal section through the hypothalamus at the level of the dorsomedial, ventromedial, and lateral hypothalamic nuclei. Lesions or stimulation of these nuclei result in obesity, cachexia, and rage. The column of the fornix separates the medial from the lateral hypothalamic zones. A lesion of the optic tract results in a contralateral hemianopia. *FX,* fornix; *DM,* medial dorsal nucleus of thalamus; *OT,* optic tract; *VL,* ventral lateral nucleus of thalamus; *VP,* ventral posterior nucleus of thalamus. (Reprinted from Fix JD. *BRS Neuroanatomy.* 3rd ed. Baltimore, MD: Williams & Wilkins; 1996:313, with permission.)

CASE 11-1

A 90-year-old woman complains of an intense burning sensation on the left side of her neck and upper limb. The patient has a history of high blood pressure and diabetes. What is the most likely diagnosis?

Differentials

- Hypoglycemia; middle cerebral artery stroke; migraine

Relevant Physical Exam Findings

- Unilateral sensory loss is observed. Though the patient may complain of weakness on the affected side, no weakness is found on examination.

Relevant Lab Findings

- Normal serum glucose levels
- Thrombocytopenia
- Ischemic infarction of posterior cerebral artery seen on computed tomography scan

Diagnosis

- Infarction of the ventral posterolateral nucleus of the thalamus results in pure hemisensory loss contralateral to the lesion.

CASE 11-2

A 65-year-old diabetic man was hospitalized after an auto accident with lethargy and progressive confusion. Laboratory tests results revealed low sodium levels. The patient was discharged after serum sodium levels were elevated to 130 mmol/L.

Differentials

- Diabetes

Relevant Physical Exam Findings

- Fatigue and depression
- Slowed mental processing time
- Slowed pulse and hypothermia
- Hyporeflexia and hypotonia

Relevant Lab Findings

- Normal hepatic, renal, and cardiac function
- Hyponatremia that worsens with fluid load
- Serum hypo-osmolality
- Urine hyperosmolarity

Diagnosis

- Inappropriate secretion of antidiuretic hormone by the hypothalamus. As many as 50% of traumatic brain injury patients experience endocrine complications that may result in intracerebral osmotic fluid shifts and brain edema, affecting hypothalamic function.

CHAPTER 12

Auditory System

Objectives

1. Describe the central and peripheral components of the auditory pathway.
2. Compare and contrast conduction and nerve deafness and describe the clinical diagnostic tests for each.
3. Outline the clinical testing and relevance of brain stem auditory evoked response (BAER).

 Introduction. The auditory system is an exteroceptive special somatic afferent system that can detect sound frequencies from 20 Hz to 20,000 Hz. It is served by the vestibulocochlear nerve (CN VIII). It is derived from the **otic vesicle,** which is a derivative of the **otic placode,** a thickening of the **surface ectoderm.**

 The Auditory Pathway (Figure 12-1) consists of the following structures:

A. The **hair cells of the organ of Corti** are innervated by the peripheral processes of bipolar cells of the spiral ganglion. They are stimulated by vibrations of the basilar membrane.

    1. Inner hair cells (IHCs) are the chief sensory elements; they synapse with dendrites of myelinated neurons whose axons make up 90% of the cochlear nerve.

    2. Outer hair cells (OHCs) synapse with dendrites of unmyelinated neurons whose axons make up 10% of the cochlear nerve. The OHCs reduce the threshold of the IHCs.

B. The **bipolar cells of the spiral (cochlear) ganglion** project peripherally to the hair cells of the organ of Corti. They project centrally as the cochlear nerve to the cochlear nuclei.

C. The **cochlear nerve (cranial nerve [CN] VIII)** extends from the spiral ganglion to the cerebellopontine angle, where it enters the brain stem.

D. The **cochlear nuclei** receive input from the cochlear nerve. They project contralaterally to the superior olivary nucleus and lateral lemniscus.

E. The **superior olivary nucleus,** which plays a role in sound localization, receives bilateral input from the cochlear nuclei. It projects to the lateral lemniscus.

F. The **trapezoid body** is located in the pons. It contains decussating fibers from the anterior cochlear nuclei.

G. The **lateral lemniscus** receives input from the contralateral cochlear nuclei and superior olivary nuclei.

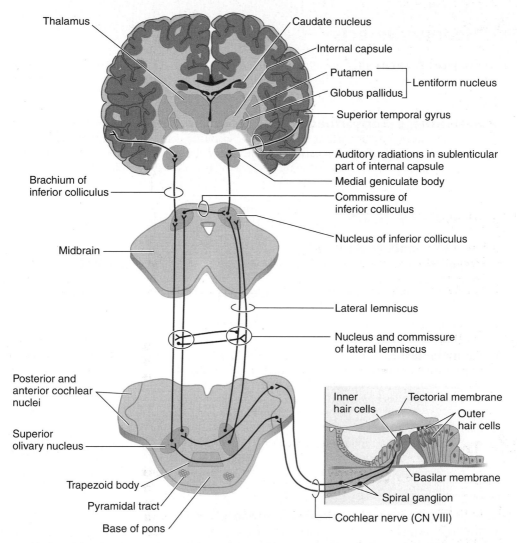

Figure 12-1 Peripheral and central connections of the auditory system. This system arises from the hair cells of the organ of Corti and terminates in the transverse temporal gyri of Heschl of the superior temporal gyrus. It is characterized by the bilaterality of projections and the tonotopic localization of pitch at all levels. For example, high pitch (20,000 Hz) is localized at the base of the cochlea and in the posteromedial part of the transverse temporal gyri. *CN,* cranial nerve.

H. The **nucleus of inferior colliculus** receives input from the lateral lemniscus. It projects through the brachium of the inferior colliculus to the medial geniculate body.

I. The **medial geniculate body** receives input from the nucleus of the inferior colliculus. It projects through the internal capsule as the auditory radiation to the primary auditory cortex, the superior temporal gyrus (transverse temporal gyri of Heschl).

J. The superior temporal gyrus **(transverse temporal gyri of Heschl)** contains the primary auditory cortex (Brodmann areas 41 and 42). The gyri are located in the depths of the **lateral sulcus.**

Hearing Defects

A. Conduction Deafness is caused by interruption of the passage of sound waves through the external or middle ear. It may be caused by **obstruction** (e.g., wax), **otosclerosis,** or **otitis media** and is often reversible.

B. Nerve Deafness (Sensorineural, or Perceptive, Deafness) is typically permanent and is caused by disease of the cochlea, cochlear nerve (acoustic neuroma), or central auditory connections. It is usually caused by **presbycusis** that results from degenerative disease of the organ of Corti in the first few millimeters of the basal coil of the cochlea (high-frequency loss of 4,000 to 8,000 Hz).

 Auditory Tests

A. Tuning Fork Tests (Table 12-1)
   1. Weber test is performed by placing a vibrating tuning fork on the vertex of the skull. Normally, a patient hears equally on both sides.
     a. A patient who has **unilateral conduction deafness** hears the vibration more loudly in the affected ear.
     b. A patient who has **unilateral partial nerve deafness** hears the vibration more loudly in the normal ear.
   2. The **Rinne test** compares air and bone conduction. It is performed by placing a vibrating tuning fork on the mastoid process until the vibration is no longer heard; then the fork is held in front of the ear. Normally, a patient hears the vibration in the air after bone conduction is gone. Note that a **positive Rinne test** means that sound conduction is normal (air conduction [AC] is greater than bone conduction [BC]), whereas a **negative Rinne test** indicates conduction loss, with BC greater than AC (Table 12-1).
     a. A patient who has **unilateral conduction deafness** does not hear the vibration in the air after bone conduction is gone.
     b. A patient who has **unilateral partial nerve deafness** hears the vibration in the air after bone conduction is gone.

B. Brain Stem Auditory Evoked Response (BAER)
   1. Testing method. Clicks are presented to one ear, then to the other. Scalp electrodes and a computer generate a series of seven waves. The waves are associated with specific areas of the auditory pathway.
   2. Diagnostic value. This method is valuable for diagnosing brain stem lesions **(multiple sclerosis)** and posterior fossa tumors **(acoustic neuromas).** It is also useful for assessing hearing in infants. Approximately 50% of patients with multiple sclerosis have abnormal BAERs.

Table 12-1: Tuning Fork Test Results

Otologic Finding	Weber Test	Rinne Test
Conduction deafness (left ear)	Lateralizes to left ear	BC > AC on left AC > BC on right
Conduction deafness (right ear)	Lateralizes to right ear	BC > AC on right AC > BC on left
Nerve deafness (left ear)	Lateralizes to right ear	AC > BC both ears
Nerve deafness (right ear)	Lateralizes to left ear	AC > BC both ears
Normal ears	No lateralization	AC > BC both ears

AC, air conduction; BC, bone conduction.

CASE 12-1

A 45-year-old woman presents with a 10-year history of auditory decline in her left ear. The problem began after her first pregnancy. There is no history of otologic infection or trauma. What is the most likely diagnosis?

Relevant Physical Exam Findings

- The external auditory meatus and tympanic membrane were benign bilaterally.
- The Weber test lateralized to the left side at 512 Hz, and the Rinne test was negative at 512 Hz on the left and was positive on the right.

Diagnosis

- Otosclerosis

CHAPTER 13

Vestibular System

Objectives

1. Differentiate between static and kinetic (dynamic) equilibrium.
2. Describe the central and peripheral components of the vestibular pathways.
3. Compare and contrast postrotational and caloric vestibular nystagmus.
4. Describe the vestibulo-ocular reflexes in the unconscious patient.

 Introduction. The vestibular system is served by the vestibulocochlear nerve (CN VIII), an SSA nerve. Like the auditory system, the vestibular system is derived from the **otic vesicle.** The otic vesicle is a derivative of the **otic placode,** which is a thickening of the **surface ectoderm.** This system maintains **posture** and **equilibrium** and coordinates **head and eye movements.**

 ## The Labyrinth

A. Kinetic Labyrinth
1. **Three semicircular ducts** lie within the three semicircular canals (i.e., superior or anterior, lateral, and posterior).
2. These ducts **respond to angular acceleration and deceleration of the head.**
   a. They contain **hair cells** in the crista ampullaris. The hair cells **respond to endolymph flow.**
   b. Endolymph flow toward the ampulla (ampullopetal) or utricle (utriculopetal) is a stronger stimulus than is endolymph flow in the opposite direction.

B. Static Labyrinth
1. The **utricle** and **saccule** respond to the position of the head with respect to **linear acceleration** and the pull of **gravity.**
2. The utricle and saccule contain **hair cells** whose cilia are embedded in the otolithic membrane. When hair cells are bent toward the longest cilium (kinocilium), the frequency of sensory discharge increases.

 ## The Vestibular Pathways (Figures 13-1 and 13-2) consist of the following structures:

A. Hair Cells of the Semicircular Ducts, Saccule, and Utricle are innervated by peripheral processes of **bipolar cells** of the vestibular ganglion.

B. The **vestibular ganglion** is located in the fundus of the internal auditory meatus.

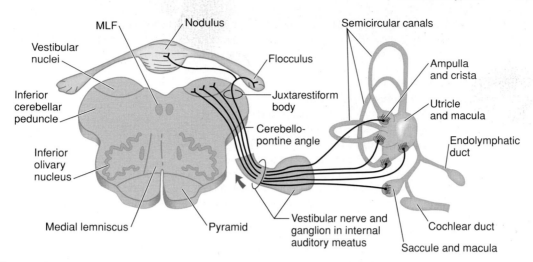

Figure 13-1 Peripheral connections of the vestibular system. The hair cells of the cristae ampullares and the maculae of the utricle and saccule project through the vestibular nerve to the vestibular nuclei of the medulla and pons and the flocculonodular lobe of the cerebellum (vestibulocerebellum). *MLF,* medial longitudinal fasciculus.

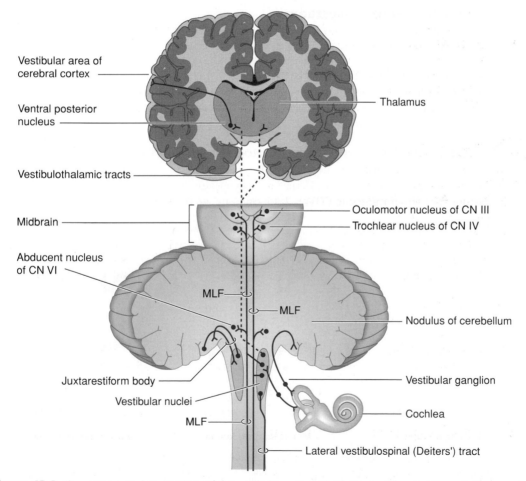

Figure 13-2 The major central connections of the vestibular system. Vestibular nuclei project through the ascending medial longitudinal fasciculi (*MLF*) to the ocular motor nuclei and subserve vestibulo-ocular reflexes. Vestibular nuclei also project through the descending MLF and lateral vestibulospinal tracts to the ventral horn motor neurons of the spinal cord and mediate postural reflexes. *CN,* cranial nerve.

1. Bipolar neurons project through their peripheral processes to the hair cells.
2. Bipolar neurons project their central processes as the vestibular nerve (cranial nerve [CN] VIII) to the vestibular nuclei and to the flocculonodular lobe of the cerebellum.

C. Vestibular Nuclei

1. **These nuclei receive input from:**
   a. The semicircular ducts, saccule, and utricle.
   b. The flocculonodular lobe of the cerebellum.
2. **The nuclei project fibers to:**
   a. The flocculonodular lobe of the cerebellum.
   b. CNs III, IV, and VI through the medial longitudinal fasciculus (MLF).
   c. The spinal cord through the lateral vestibulospinal tract.
   d. The ventral posteroinferior and posterolateral nuclei of the thalamus, both of which project to the postcentral gyrus.

IV Vestibulo-ocular Reflexes are mediated by the vestibular nuclei, MLF, ocular motor nuclei, and CNs III, IV, and VI.

A. Vestibular (Horizontal) Nystagmus

1. The **fast phase** of nystagmus is in the **direction of rotation.**
2. The **slow phase** of nystagmus is in the **opposite direction.**

B. Postrotatory (Horizontal) Nystagmus

1. The **fast phase** of nystagmus is in the **opposite direction of rotation.**
2. The **slow phase** of nystagmus is in the **direction of rotation.**
3. The patient past-points and falls in the direction of previous rotation.

C. Caloric Nystagmus (Stimulation of Horizontal Ducts) in normal subjects

1. **Cold water irrigation** of the external auditory meatus results in nystagmus to the opposite side.
2. **Warm water irrigation** of the external auditory meatus results in nystagmus to the same side.
3. **Remember the mnemonic COWS: c**old, **o**pposite, **w**arm, **s**ame.

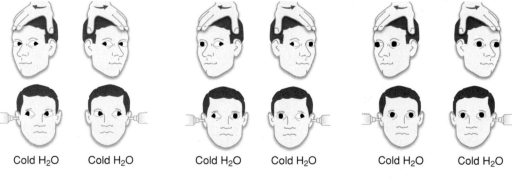

Figure 13-3 Ocular reflexes in comatose patients. The external auditory meatus is irrigated with cold water. If the brainstem is intact, the eyes deviate toward the irrigated side. If the MLFs are transected, the eyes deviate toward the side of the abducted eye only. With lower brainstem damage, the eyes do not deviate from the midline. (Adapted with permission from Plum F, Posner GB. *The Diagnosis of Stupor and Coma.* 3rd ed. Philadelphia, PA: FA Davis; 1982:55.)

D. Test Results in **Unconscious Subjects** (Figure 13-3)

    1. No nystagmus is seen in normal conscious subjects.

    2. When the brain stem is intact, there is deviation of the eyes to the side of the cold irrigation in unconscious subjects.

    3. With bilateral MLF transaction in unconscious subjects, there is deviation of the abducting eye to the side of the cold irrigation.

    4. With lower brain stem damage to the vestibular nuclei, there is no deviation of the eyes in unconscious subjects.

CASE 13-1

A 60-year-old woman came to the clinic with complaints of progressive hearing loss, facial weakness, and headaches on the right side. She also said that she had become more unsteady in walking, with weakness and numbness of the right side of the face. No nausea or vomiting was noted. What is the most likely diagnosis?

Relevant Physical Exam Findings

- Reduced pain and touch sensation in right face
- Right facial weakness
- Absent right corneal reflex
- Hearing loss on right side
- No response to caloric test stimulation on right side
- Bilateral papilledema

Diagnosis

- Acoustic neuroma

CHAPTER 14

Visual System

Objectives

1. Outline the central and peripheral components of the visual pathway.
2. List the retinal layers and cell types found in each layer.
3. Describe the result of lesions at the optic nerve, optic chiasm, and optic tract.
4. Compare and contrast the pupillary reflexes, including direct versus consensual reflexes, dilation, convergence, and accommodation.
5. Summarize the various clinical correlates related to the visual system.

 Introduction. The visual system is served by the optic nerve, which is a special somatic afferent (SSA) nerve.

 The Visual Pathway (Figure 14-1) includes the following structures:

A. Ganglion Cells of the Retina form the optic nerve (cranial nerve [CN] II). They project from the nasal hemiretina to the contralateral lateral geniculate body and from the temporal hemiretina to the ipsilateral lateral geniculate body.

B. The **optic nerve** projects from the lamina cribrosa of the scleral canal, through the optic canal, to the optic chiasm (Figure 14-2).
   1. **Transection of the optic nerve** causes ipsilateral blindness, with no direct pupillary light reflex.
   2. A lesion of the optic nerve at the optic chiasm transects all fibers from the ipsilateral retina and fibers from the contralateral inferior nasal quadrant that loop into the optic nerve. This **lesion** causes ipsilateral blindness and a contralateral upper temporal quadrant defect **(junction scotoma).**

C. The **optic chiasm** contains decussating fibers from the two nasal hemiretinas. It contains noncrossing fibers from the two temporal hemiretinas and projects fibers to the suprachiasmatic nucleus of the hypothalamus.
   1. **Midsagittal transection or pressure** (often from a pituitary tumor) causes bitemporal hemianopia.
   2. **Bilateral lateral compression** causes binasal hemianopia (often from calcified internal carotid arteries).

D. The **optic tract** contains fibers from the ipsilateral temporal hemiretina and the contralateral nasal hemiretina. It projects to the ipsilateral lateral geniculate body, pretectal nuclei, and superior colliculus. Transection causes contralateral hemianopia.

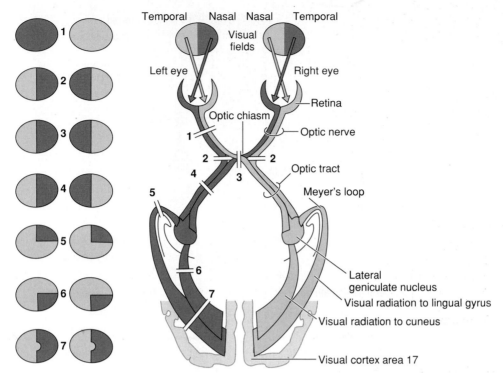

Temporal   Nasal Nasal   Temporal

Visual fields

Left eye   Right eye

Retina

Optic chiasm

Optic nerve

Optic tract

Meyer's loop

Lateral geniculate nucleus

Visual radiation to lingual gyrus

Visual radiation to cuneus

Visual cortex area 17

Figure 14-1 The visual pathway from the retina to the visual cortex showing visual field defects. (1) Ipsilateral blindness. (2) Binasal hemianopia. (3) Bitemporal hemianopia. (4) Right hemianopia. (5) Right upper quadrantanopia. (6) Right lower quadrantanopia. (7) Right hemianopia with macular sparing. (8) Left constricted field as a result of end-stage glaucoma. Bilateral constricted fields may be seen in hysteria. (9) Left central scotoma as seen in optic (retrobulbar) neuritis in multiple sclerosis. (10) Upper altitudinal hemianopia as a result of bilateral destruction of the lingual gyri. (11) Lower altitudinal hemianopia as a result of bilateral destruction of the cunei.

E. The **lateral geniculate body** is a six-layered nucleus. Layers 1, 4, and 6 receive crossed fibers; layers 2, 3, and 5 receive uncrossed fibers. The lateral geniculate body receives input from layer VI of the striate cortex (Brodmann area 17). It also receives fibers from the ipsilateral temporal hemiretina and the contralateral nasal hemiretina. It projects through the geniculocalcarine tract to layer IV of the primary visual cortex (Brodmann area 17).

F. The **geniculocalcarine tract (visual radiation)** projects through two divisions to the visual cortex.
  1. The **upper division** (Figure 14-3) projects to the upper bank of the calcarine sulcus, the cuneus. It contains input from the superior retinal quadrants, which represent the inferior visual field quadrants.
    a. Transection causes a contralateral lower quadrantanopia.
    b. Lesions that involve both cunei cause a lower altitudinal hemianopia (altitudinopia).
  2. The **lower division** (see Figure 14-3) loops from the lateral geniculate body anteriorly (Meyer loop), then posteriorly, to terminate in the lower bank of the calcarine sulcus, the lingual gyrus. It contains input from the inferior retinal quadrants, which represent the superior visual field quadrants.
    a. Transection causes a **contralateral upper quadrantanopia** ("pie in the sky").
    b. Transection of both lingual gyri causes an **upper altitudinal hemianopia (altitudinopia).**

G. The **visual cortex (Brodmann area 17)** is located on the banks of the calcarine fissure. The **cuneus** is the upper bank. The **lingual gyrus** is the lower bank. Lesions cause **contralateral hemianopia** with macular sparing. The visual cortex has a **retinotopic organization:**
  1. The **posterior area** receives macular input (central vision).
  2. The **intermediate area** receives paramacular input (peripheral input).
  3. The **anterior area** receives monocular input.

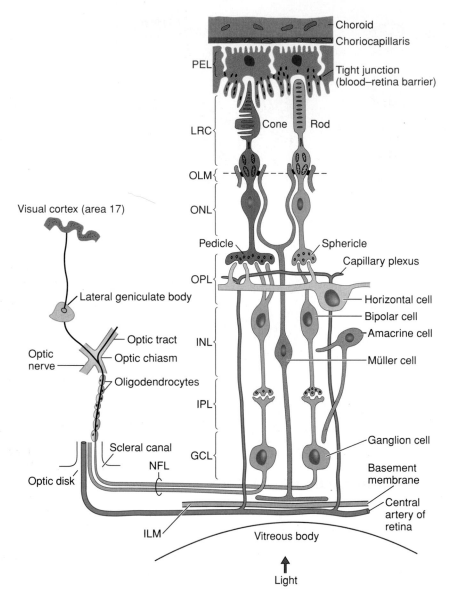

Figure 14-2 Histology of the retina. The retina has ten layers: (1) pigment epithelium layer (*PEL*), (2) layer of rods and cones (*LRC*), (3) outer limiting membrane (*OLM*), (4) outer nuclear layer (*ONL*), (5) outer plexiform layer (*OPL*), (6) inner nuclear layer (*INL*), (7) inner plexiform layer (*IPL*), (8) ganglion cell layer (*GCL*), (9) nerve fiber layer (*NFL*), and (10) inner limiting layer (*ILL*). The tight junctions binding the pigment epithelial cells make up the blood–retina barrier. Retinal detachment usually occurs between the pigment layer and the layer of rods and cones. The central artery of the retina perfuses the retina to the outer plexiform layer, and the choriocapillaris supplies the outer five layers of the retina. The Müller cells are radial glial cells that have support function. Myelin of the central nervous system (CNS) is produced by oligodendrocytes, which are not normally found in the retina. (Adapted from Dudek RW. *High-Yield Histology*. Baltimore, MD: Williams & Wilkins; 1997:64, with permission.)

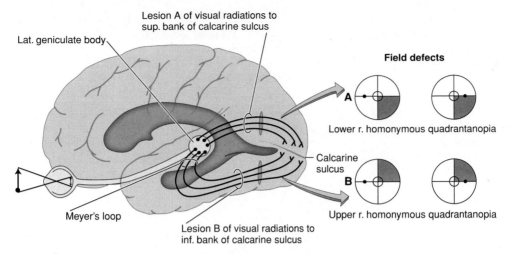

Lesion A of visual radiations to
sup. bank of calcarine sulcus

Lat. geniculate body

Field defects

A

Lower r. homonymous quadrantanopia

Calcarine
sulcus

B

Meyer's loop

Upper r. homonymous quadrantanopia

Lesion B of visual radiations to
inf. bank of calcarine sulcus

Figure 14-3 Relations of the left upper and left lower divisions of the geniculocalcarine tract to the lateral ventricle and calcarine sulcus. Transection of the upper division **(A)** results in right lower homonymous quadrantanopia. Transection of the lower division **(B)** results in right upper homonymous quadrantanopia. (Reprinted from Fix JD. *BRS Neuroanatomy*. Baltimore, MD: Williams & Wilkins; 1997:261, with permission.)

III The Pupillary Light Reflex Pathway (Figure 14-4) has an afferent
limb (CN II) and an efferent limb (CN III). It includes the following structures:

A. Ganglion Cells of the Retina, which project bilaterally to the pretectal nuclei.

B. The **pretectal nucleus of the midbrain,** which projects (through the posterior commissure) crossed and uncrossed fibers to the accessory oculomotor (Edinger–Westphal) nucleus.

C. The **accessory oculomotor** (Edinger–Westphal) **nucleus of CN III,** which gives rise to preganglionic parasympathetic fibers. These fibers exit the midbrain with CN III and synapse with postganglionic parasympathetic neurons of the ciliary ganglion.

D. The **ciliary ganglion,** which gives rise to postganglionic parasympathetic fibers. These fibers innervate the sphincter pupillae.

IV The Pupillary Dilation Pathway (Figure 14-5) is mediated by the
sympathetic division of the autonomic nervous system. Interruption of this pathway at any level causes ipsilateral **Horner syndrome.** It includes the following structures:

A. The **hypothalamus**. Hypothalamic neurons of the paraventricular nucleus project directly to the **ciliospinal center** (T1–T2) of the intermediolateral cell column of the spinal cord.

B. The **ciliospinal center** of Budge **(T1–T2)** projects preganglionic sympathetic fibers through the sympathetic trunk to the superior cervical ganglion.

C. The **superior cervical ganglion** projects postganglionic sympathetic fibers through the perivascular plexus of the carotid system to the dilator muscle of the iris. Postganglionic sympathetic fibers pass through the **tympanic cavity** and **cavernous sinus** and enter the orbit through the **superior orbital fissure.**

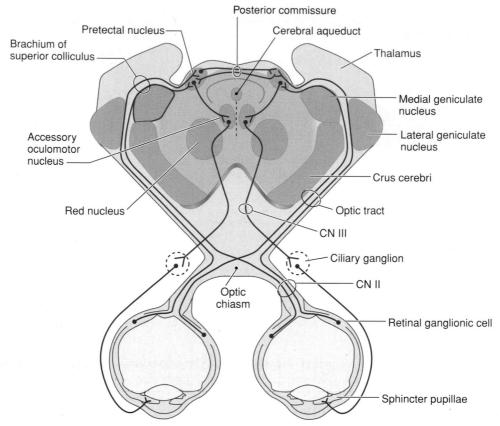

Figure 14-4 The pupillary light pathway. Light shined into one eye causes both pupils to constrict. The response in the stimulated eye is called the *direct pupillary light reflex.* The response in the opposite eye is called the *consensual pupillary light reflex. CN,* cranial nerve.

 The Near Reflex and Accommodation Pathway

A. The **cortical visual pathway** projects from the primary visual cortex (Brodmann area 17) to the visual association cortex (Brodmann area 19).

B. The **visual association cortex (Brodmann area 19)** projects through the corticotectal tract to the superior colliculus and pretectal nucleus.

C. The **superior colliculus** and **pretectal nucleus** project to the **oculomotor complex** of the **midbrain.** This complex includes the following structures:
   1. The **rostral accessory oculomotor** (Edinger–Westphal) **nucleus,** which mediates pupillary constriction through the ciliary ganglion.
   2. The **caudal accessory oculomotor** (Edinger–Westphal) **nucleus,** which mediates contraction of the ciliary muscle. This contraction increases the refractive power of the lens.
   3. The **medial rectus subnucleus of CN III (nucleus of Perlia)** which mediates convergence.

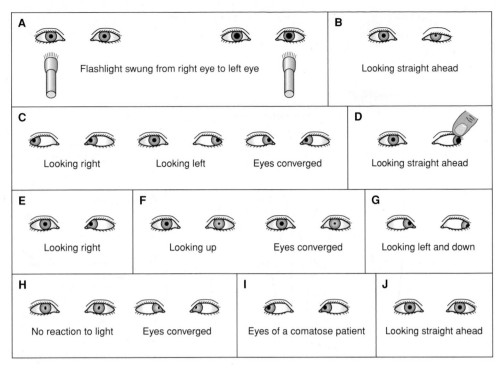

Figure 14-5 Ocular motor palsies and pupillary syndromes. **A.** Relative afferent (Marcus Gunn) pupil, left eye. **B.** Horner syndrome, left eye. **C.** Internuclear ophthalmoplegia, right eye. **D.** Third-nerve palsy, left eye. **E.** Sixth-nerve palsy, right eye. **F.** Paralysis of upward gaze and convergence (Parinaud syndrome). **G.** Fourth-nerve palsy, right eye. **H.** Argyll Robertson pupil. **I.** Destructive lesion of the right frontal eye field. **J.** Third-nerve palsy with ptosis, right eye.

 VI   Cortical and Subcortical Centers for Ocular Motility

A. The **frontal eye field** is located in the posterior part of the middle frontal gyrus (Brodmann area 8). It regulates voluntary (saccadic) eye movements.

    1. Stimulation (e.g., from an irritative lesion) causes **contralateral deviation of the eyes** (i.e., away from the lesion).

    2. Destruction causes **transient ipsilateral conjugate deviation of the eyes** (i.e., toward the lesion).

B. Occipital Eye Fields are located in Brodmann areas 18 and 19 of the occipital lobes. These fields are cortical centers for involuntary (smooth) pursuit and tracking movements. **Stimulation** causes contralateral conjugate deviation of the eyes.

C. The **subcortical center for lateral conjugate gaze** is located in the paramedian pontine reticular formation (Figure 14-6).

    1. It receives input from the contralateral frontal eye field.

    2. It projects to the ipsilateral lateral rectus muscle and through the medial longitudinal fasciculus (MLF) to the contralateral medial rectus subnucleus of the oculomotor complex.

D. The **subcortical center for vertical conjugate gaze** is located in the midbrain at the level of the posterior commissure. It is called the *rostral interstitial nucleus* of the MLF and is associated with **Parinaud syndrome** (see Figure 14-5F).

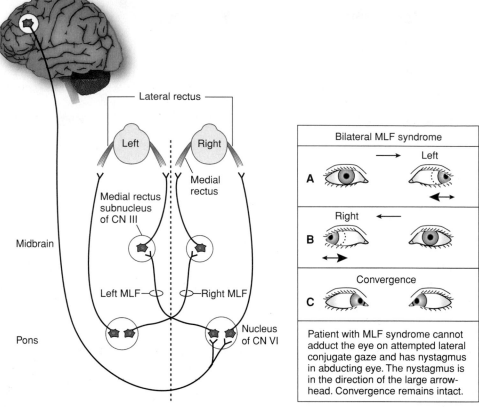

Figure 14-6 Connections of the pontine center for lateral conjugate gaze. Lesions of the medial longitudinal fasciculus (*MLF*) between the abducent and oculomotor nuclei result in medial rectus palsy on attempted lateral conjugate gaze and horizontal nystagmus in the abducting eye. Convergence remains intact (*inset*). A unilateral MLF lesion would affect only the ipsilateral medial rectus. *CN,* cranial nerve.

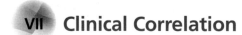 **Clinical Correlation**

A. In **MLF syndrome,** or **internuclear ophthalmoplegia** (see Figure 14-5), there is damage (demyelination) to the MLF between the abducent and oculomotor nuclei. It causes **medial rectus palsy on attempted lateral conjugate gaze** and monocular horizontal nystagmus in the abducting eye. **(Convergence is normal.)** This syndrome is most commonly seen in **multiple sclerosis.**

B. One-and-a-half Syndrome consists of bilateral lesions of the MLF and a unilateral lesion of the abducent nucleus. On attempted lateral conjugate gaze, the only muscle that functions is the intact lateral rectus.

C. Argyll Robertson Pupil (pupillary light–near dissociation) is the absence of a miotic reaction to light, both direct and consensual, with the preservation of a miotic reaction to near stimulus (accommodation–convergence). It occurs in **syphilis, diabetes mellitus, and lupus erythematosus.**

D. Horner Syndrome is caused by transection of the oculosympathetic pathway at any level. This syndrome consists of miosis, ptosis, apparent enophthalmos, and hemianhidrosis.

E. Afferent (Marcus Gunn) Pupil results from a lesion of the optic nerve, the afferent limb of the pupillary light reflex (e.g., retrobulbar neuritis seen in multiple sclerosis). The diagnosis can be made with the swinging flashlight test (see Figure 14-5A).

F. Transtentorial (Uncal) Herniation occurs as a result of **increased supratentorial pressure,** which is commonly caused by a brain tumor or hematoma (subdural or epidural).

   1. The pressure cone forces the parahippocampal uncus through the tentorial incisure.

   2. The impacted uncus forces the contralateral crus cerebri against the tentorial edge (Kernohan notch) and puts pressure on the ipsilateral CN III and posterior cerebral artery. As a result, the following neurologic defects occur:

      a. Ipsilateral hemiparesis occurs as a result of pressure on the corticospinal tract, which is located in the contralateral crus cerebri.

      b. A **fixed and dilated pupil, ptosis,** and a **"down-and-out" eye** are caused by pressure on the ipsilateral oculomotor nerve.

      c. Contralateral homonymous hemianopia is caused by compression of the posterior cerebral artery, which irrigates the visual cortex.

G. Papilledema (Choked Disk) is noninflammatory congestion of the optic disk as a result of increased intracranial pressure. It is most commonly caused by brain tumors, subdural hematoma, or hydrocephalus. It usually **does not alter visual acuity,** but it may cause bilateral **enlarged blind spots.** It is often asymmetric and is greater on the side of the supratentorial lesion.

H. Adie (Holmes-Adie) Pupil is a large tonic pupil that reacts slowly to light but does react to near (light–near dissociation). It is frequently seen in women with absent knee or ankle jerks.

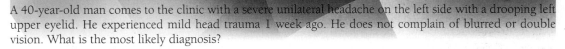

CASE 14-1

A 40-year-old man comes to the clinic with a severe unilateral headache on the left side with a drooping left upper eyelid. He experienced mild head trauma 1 week ago. He does not complain of blurred or double vision. What is the most likely diagnosis?

Relevant Physical Exam Findings

- The right pupil is 4 mm and normally reactive, and the left pupil is 2 mm and normally reactive.
- The left pupil dilates poorly.
- There is 2- to 3-mm ptosis of the left upper eyelid.

Diagnosis

- Horner's syndrome

CHAPTER 15

Limbic System

Objectives

1. List the components of the limbic system.
2. Describe the major fiber pathways associated with the limbic system, include their targets.
3. Define the major causes and symptoms associated with damage to the hippocampus and the amygdala.
4. Describe Klüver–Bucy syndrome, Wernicke encephalopathy, and Papez Circuit.

 Introduction. The limbic system is responsible for the consolidation of short-term memories into long and is considered the anatomic substrate that underlies behavior and emotional expression—through the hypothalamus by way of the autonomic nervous system.

 ## Major Components

A. The **medial and basal forebrain** contains the **septal area** and **ventral striatum,** which functions in behavior and emotional states and the reward/punishment system. The septal area is reciprocally connected to the hypothalamus via the fornix, to the hypothalamus via the **medial forebrain bundle** and the **habenula** via the **stria terminalis.** The **ventral** forebrain is positioned to affect posture and muscle tone that accompany behavior and emotional states.

B. The **hippocampal formation** is composed of the hippocampus proper, dentate gyrus, and subiculum. It is connected reciprocally to the entorhinal cortex and septum via the fornix, and to the mammillary bodies of the hypothalamus via the fornix. The medial temporal lobe components are involved in recognition of novelty and in memory consolidation.

C. The **limbic lobe,** composed of the cingulate gyrus and medial temporal lobe, contains the **parahippocampal gyrus** and the **amygdala** (Figure 15-1). It is involved in the emotional response to stimuli and in memory consolidation.

 ## The Papez Circuit (Figure 15-2) includes the following limbic structures:

A. The **hippocampal formation,** which projects through the fornix to the mammillary bodies and septal area

B. The **mammillary bodies**

C. The **anterior thalamic nucleus**

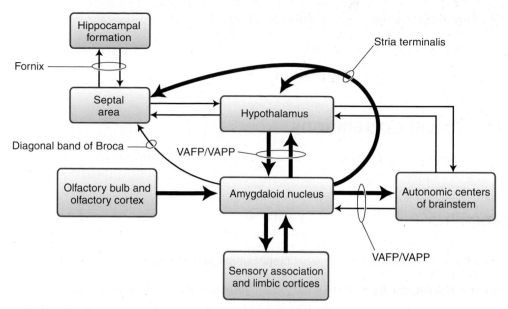

Figure 15-1 Major connections of the amygdaloid nucleus. This nucleus receives input from three major sources: the olfactory system, sensory association and limbic cortices, and hypothalamus. Major output is through two channels: the stria terminalis projects to the hypothalamus and the septal area, and the ventral amygdalofugal pathway (*VAFP*) projects to the hypothalamus, brain stem, and spinal cord. A smaller efferent bundle, the diagonal band of Broca, projects to the septal area. Afferent fibers from the hypothalamus and brain stem enter the amygdaloid nucleus through the ventral amygdalopetal pathway (*VAPP*).

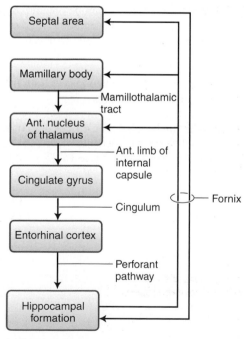

Figure 15-2 Major afferent and efferent limbic connections of the hippocampal formation. This formation has three components: the hippocampus (cornu ammonis), subiculum, and dentate gyrus. The hippocampus projects to the septal area, the subiculum projects to the mammillary nuclei, and the dentate gyrus does not project beyond the hippocampal formation. The circuit of Papez follows this route: hippocampal formation to mammillary nucleus to anterior thalamic nucleus to cingulate gyrus to entorhinal cortex to hippocampal formation.

D. The **cingulate gyrus** (Brodmann areas 23 and 24)

E. The **entorhinal area** (Brodmann area 28)

F. Back to the **hippocampal formation**

 IV Clinical Correlations

A. Klüver–Bucy Syndrome results from bilateral ablation of the anterior temporal lobes, to include the amygdaloid nuclei. It causes psychic blindness (visual agnosia), hyperphagia, docility (placidity), and hypersexuality.

B. Amnestic (Confabulatory) Syndrome results from bilateral infarction of the hippocampal formation (i.e., hippocampal branches of the posterior cerebral arteries and anterior choroidal arteries of the internal carotid arteries). It causes anterograde amnesia (i.e., inability to learn and retain new information). **Memory loss** suggests **hippocampal pathology.**

C. Foster Kennedy Syndrome results from **meningioma** of the **olfactory groove.** The meningioma compresses the olfactory tract and optic nerve. Ipsilateral anosmia and optic atrophy and contralateral papilledema occur as a result of increased intracranial pressure.

D. The **hippocampus** is the most epileptogenic part of the cerebrum. Lesions may cause psychomotor attacks. Sommer sector is very sensitive to ischemia.

E. Bilateral transection of the fornix may cause the acute amnestic syndrome (i.e., inability to consolidate short-term memory into long-term memory).

F. Wernicke Encephalopathy results from a thiamine (vitamin B_1) deficiency. The clinical triad includes ocular disturbances and nystagmus, gait ataxia, and mental dysfunction. Pathologic features include mammillary nuclei (bodies), dorsomedial nuclei of the thalamus, periaqueductal gray, and the pontine tegmentum.

G. Strachan Syndrome results from high-dose thiamine (vitamin B_1) therapy. The clinical triad includes spinal ataxia, optic atrophy, and nerve deafness.

H. Bilateral destruction or removal of the cingulate gyri causes loss of initiative and inhibition and dulling of the emotions. Memory is unaffected. Lesions of the anterior cingulate gyri cause placidity. Cingulectomy is used to treat severe anxiety and depression (Figure 15-3).

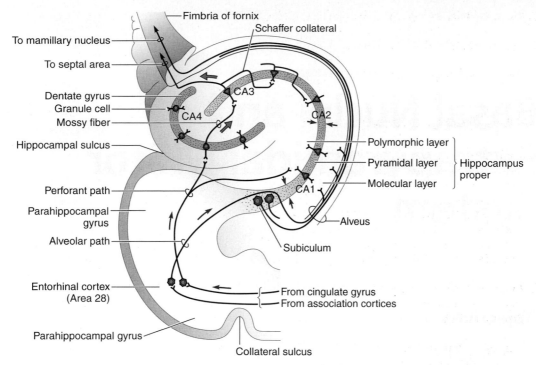

Figure 15-3 Major connections of the hippocampal formation. The hippocampal formation (HF) consists of three parts: hippocampus, dentate gyrus, and subiculum. The two major hypothalamic output pathways are (1) granule cell via mossy fiber to pyramidal cell via precommissural fornix to septal nuclei and (2) subicular neuron via postcommissural fornix to the medial mammillary nucleus. The HF plays an important role in learning and memory, and lesions of the HF result in short-term memory defects. In Alzheimer disease, loss of cells in the HF and entorhinal cortex leads to loss of memory and cognitive function. *CA,* cornu ammonis. The sector CA1 is very sensitive to hypoxia (cardiac arrest or stroke). (Reprinted from Fix JD. *BRS Neuroanatomy.* 3rd ed. Baltimore, MD: Williams & Wilkins; 1996:332, with permission.)

CASE 15-1

A 15-year-old boy was knocked out after several rounds of boxing with friends. Computed tomography scanning showed acute subdural hematoma associated with the right cerebral hemisphere. After regaining consciousness, the boy no longer experienced normal fear and anger and demonstrated aberrant sexual behaviors and excessive oral tendencies. He also complained of being very hungry all the time. What is the most likely diagnosis?

Relevant Lab Findings

● Computed tomography and magnetic resonance imaging revealed lesions of the right temporal lobe and right-dominant orbitofrontal regions, including bilateral rectal and medial orbital gyri, and an intact left temporal lobe.

Diagnosis

● Klüver-Bucy syndrome occurs when both the right and left medial temporal lobes malfunction, with frequent involvement of the amygdala. The cardinal symptom is excessive oral tendencies where the patient puts all types of objects into the mouth. Such patients also have an irresistible impulse to touch objects and demonstrate placidity (lack of emotional response) and a marked increase in sexual activity, without concern for social appropriateness.

CHAPTER 16

Basal Nuclei and Extrapyramidal Motor System

Objectives

1. List the components of the basal nuclei.
2. Define striatum, corpus striatum, and claustrum.
3. Describe the anatomical structures that make up the extrapyramidal system and outline their functions.
4. Describe the anatomy, clinical signs, and treatment of Parkinson Disease, Huntington Disease, hemiballism, Wilson Disease, and tardive dyskinesia.

 I   Basal Nuclei (Ganglia) (Figure 16-1)

A. Components
1. **Caudate nucleus**
2. **Putamen**
3. **Globus pallidus**

B. Grouping of the Basal Nuclei
1. The **striatum** consists of the caudate nucleus and putamen.
2. The **lentiform nucleus** consists of the globus pallidus and putamen.
3. The **corpus striatum** consists of the lentiform nucleus and caudate nucleus.
4. The **claustrum** lies between the lentiform nucleus and the insular cortex. It has reciprocal connections between the sensory cortices (i.e., visual cortex) (Figures 16-2 to 16-4).

 II   The Extrapyramidal (Striatal) Motor System (see Figure 16-1) plays a role in the initiation and execution of somatic motor activity, especially willed movement. It is also involved in automatic stereotyped postural and reflex motor activity (e.g., normal subjects swing their arms when they walk).

A. Structure. The striatal motor system includes the following structures:
1. **Neocortex**
2. **Striatum (caudatoputamen or neostriatum)**

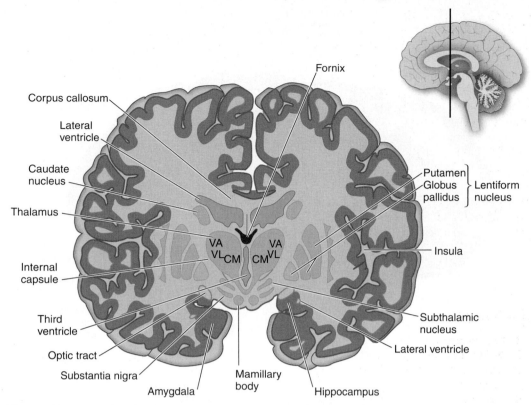

Figure 16-1 Coronal section through the midthalamus at the level of the mammillary bodies. The basal nuclei (ganglia) are all prominent at this level and include the striatum and lentiform nucleus. The subthalamic nucleus and substantia nigra are important components of the striatal motor system. *CM,* centromedian nucleus; *VA,* ventral anterior nucleus; *VL,* ventral lateral nucleus.

3. **Globus pallidus**
4. **Subthalamic nucleus**
5. **Substantia nigra** (i.e., pars compacta and pars reticularis)
6. **Thalamus** (ventral anterior, ventral lateral, and centromedian nuclei)

B. Figure 16-5 shows the **major afferent** and **efferent connections** of the striatal system.

C. Neurotransmitters are seen in Figure 16-6.

III Clinical Correlation

A. Parkinson Disease. This is a **degenerative disease** that affects the substantia nigra and its projections to the striatum.

1. **Results** of Parkinson disease are a **depletion of dopamine** in the substantia nigra and striatum as well as a **loss of melanin-containing dopaminergic neurons** in the substantia nigra.
2. **Clinical signs** are bradykinesia, stooped posture, shuffling gait, cogwheel rigidity, pill-rolling tremor, and masked facies. **Lewy bodies** are found in the melanin-containing neurons of the substantia nigra. **Progressive supranuclear palsy** is associated with Parkinson disease.
3. **Treatment** has been successful with L-dopa. Surgical intervention includes **pallidotomy** (rigidity) and **ventral thalamotomy** (tremor).

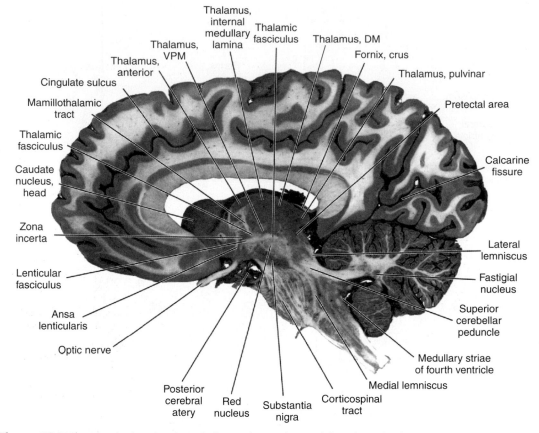

Figure 16-2 A parasagittal section through the caudate nucleus and the substantia nigra.

B. Methylphenyltetrahydropyridine (MPTP)-induced Parkinsonism. MPTP is an analog of meperidine (Demerol). It destroys dopaminergic neurons in the substantia nigra.

C. Huntington Disease (chorea). This is an **inherited autosomal dominant movement disorder** that is traced to a single gene defect on chromosome 4.
1. It is associated with **degeneration of the cholinergic and g-aminobutyric acid (GABA)-ergic neurons** of the striatum. It is accompanied by gyral atrophy in the frontal and temporal lobes.
2. **Glutamate (GLU) excitotoxicity** results when GLU is released in the striatum and binds to its receptors on striatal neurons, culminating in an action potential. GLU is removed from the extracellular space by astrocytes. In Huntington disease, GLU is bound to the N-methyl-D-aspartate receptor, resulting in an influx of calcium ions and subsequent cell death. This cascade of events with neuronal death most likely occurs in cerebrovascular accidents (e.g., stroke).
3. **Clinical signs** include choreiform movements, hypotonia, and progressive dementia.

D. Other Choreiform Dyskinesias
1. **Sydenham chorea (St. Vitus dance)** is the most common cause of chorea overall. It occurs primarily in girls, typically after a bout of rheumatic fever.
2. **Chorea gravidarum** usually occurs during the second trimester of pregnancy. Many patients have a history of Sydenham chorea.

E. Hemiballism is a **movement disorder** that usually results from a vascular lesion of the subthalamic nucleus. Clinical signs include violent contralateral **flinging (ballistic) movements of one or both extremities.**

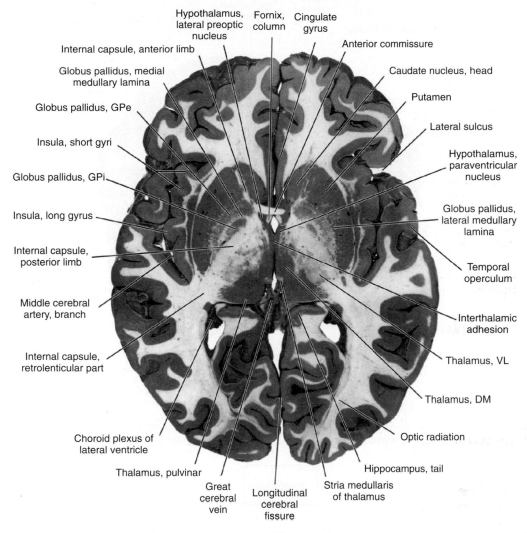

Figure 16-3 An axial (horizontal) section through the anterior commissure and the massa intermedia.

F. Hepatolenticular Degeneration (Wilson Disease) is an autosomal recessive disorder that is caused by a defect in the **metabolism of copper.** The gene locus is on chromosome 13.

1. **Clinical signs** include choreiform or athetotic movements, rigidity, and **wing-beating tremor.** Tremor is the most common neurologic sign.

2. **Lesions** are found in the **lentiform nucleus.** Copper deposition in the limbus of the cornea gives rise to the **corneal Kayser–Fleischer ring,** which is a pathognomonic sign. Deposition of copper in the liver leads to multilobular cirrhosis.

3. **Psychiatric symptoms** include psychosis, personality disorders, and dementia.

4. The **diagnosis** is based on low serum ceruloplasmin, elevated urinary excretion of copper, and increased copper concentration in a liver biopsy specimen.

5. **Treatment** includes **penicillamine,** a **chelator.**

G. Tardive Dyskinesia is a syndrome of **repetitive choreic movement** that **affects the face and trunk.** It results from treatment with phenothiazines, butyrophenones, or metoclopramide.

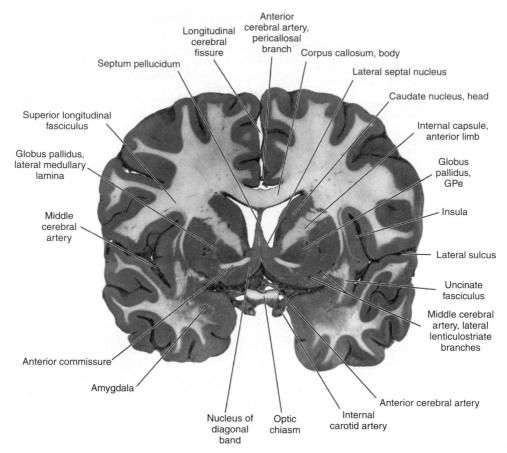

Figure 16-4 A coronal section through the lentiform nucleus and the amygdaloid nucleus; the lentiform nucleus consists of the putamen and the globus pallidus; the amygdaloid nucleus appears as a circular profile below the uncus.

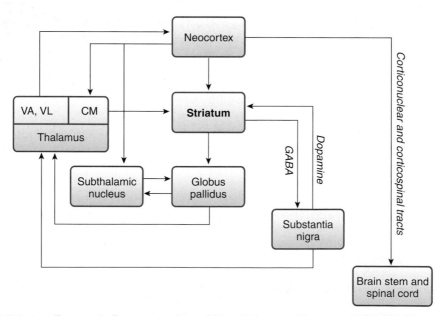

Figure 16-5 Major afferent and efferent connections of the striatal system. The striatum receives major input from three sources: the thalamus, neocortex, and substantia nigra. The striatum projects to the globus pallidus and substantia nigra. The globus pallidus is the effector nucleus of the striatal system; it projects to the thalamus and subthalamic nucleus. The substantia nigra also projects to the thalamus. The striatal motor system is expressed through the corticonuclear and cortico-spinal tracts. *CM*, centromedian nucleus; *GABA*, γ-aminobutyric acid; *VA*, ventral anterior nucleus; *VL*, ventral lateral nucleus.

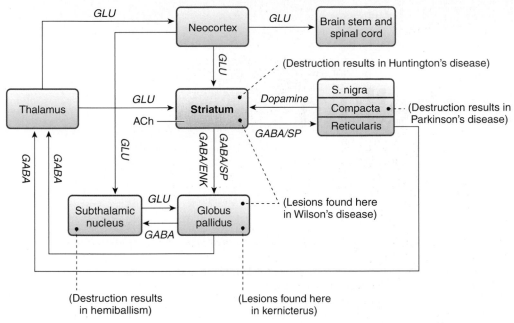

Figure 16-6 Major neurotransmitters of the extrapyramidal motor system. Within the striatum, globus pallidus, and pars reticularis of the substantia nigra (*S. nigra*), γ-aminobutyric acid (*GABA*) is the predominant neurotransmitter. GABA may coexist in the same neuron with enkephalin (*ENK*) or substance P (*SP*). Dopamine-containing neurons are found in the pars compacta of the substantia nigra. Acetylcholine (*ACh*) is found in the local circuit neurons of the striatum. The subthalamic nucleus projects excitatory glutaminergic fibers to the globus pallidus. *GLU,* glutamate.

CASE 16-1

A 30-year-old man presents with dysarthria, dysphagia, stiffness, and slow ataxic gait. There is no history of schizophrenia or depression and no family history of any neurodegenerative disease.

Relevant Physical Exam Findings

- The patient scored a 20/26 on the mini-mental status exam. The patient showed increased tone in all extremities, with normal strength.

Relevant Lab Findings

- A generalized cerebral and cerebellar atrophy and a very small caudate nucleus were revealed on magnetic resonance imaging scans.

Diagnosis

- Huntington disease (chorea) is caused by a trinucleotide repeat in the gene coding for the Huntingtin protein. It is characterized by abnormal body movements and lack of coordination but can also affect mental abilities.

CHAPTER 17

Cerebellum

Objectives

1. Be able to identify the cerebellar peduncles as to their location and relationships and describe the main contents of each.
2. Describe the cerebellar cortex and be able to identify the major cell types found in each layer.
3. Describe the Purkinje cell and its connections.
4. Identify the deep cerebellar nuclei and their output targets.
5. Assess the result(s) of cerebellar dysfunction and describe the symptoms associated with cerebellar syndromes and disorders.

 Function. The cerebellum has three primary functions:

A. Maintenance of Posture and Balance

B. Maintenance of Muscle Tone

C. Coordination of Voluntary Motor Activity

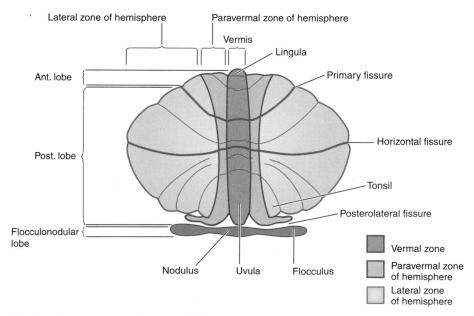

Figure 17-1 Longitudinal divisions of the cerebellum.

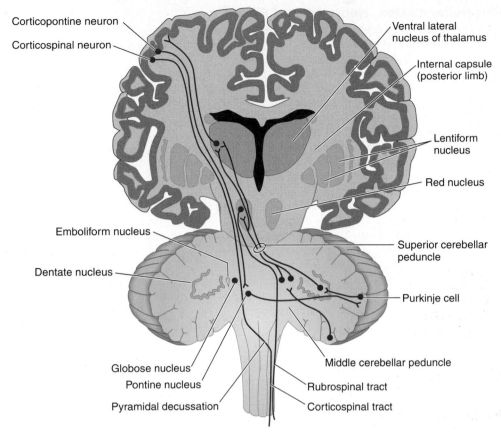

Corticopontine neuron

Corticospinal neuron

Ventral lateral
nucleus of thalamus

Internal capsule
(posterior limb)

Lentiform
nucleus

Red nucleus

Emboliform nucleus

Superior cerebellar
peduncle

Dentate nucleus

Purkinje cell

Globose nucleus

Middle cerebellar peduncle

Pontine nucleus

Rubrospinal tract

Pyramidal decussation

Corticospinal tract

Figure 17-2 The principal cerebellar connections. The major efferent pathway is the dentatothalamocortical tract. The cerebellum receives input from the cerebral cortex through the corticopontocerebellar tract.

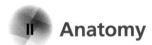 **Anatomy**

A. Gross anatomically, the cerebellum may be divided longitudinally into **lobes**, or laterally into **zones** (Figure 17-1).

1. Longitudinally the primary fissure forms an anterior lobe and posterior lobe. The posterolateral fissure separates a flocculonodular lobe from the more anterior posterior lobe (Figure 17-1).

2. Laterally the cerebellum is divided into a large lateral zone or hemisphere, a smaller intermediate (or paravermal) zone and a midline vermal zone (Figure 17-2).

B. Cerebellar Peduncles

1. The **superior cerebellar peduncle** is attached to the brainstem at the caudal midbrain and rostral pons and it contains the major output from the cerebellum, the dentatothalamic tract. This tract terminates in the ventral lateral nucleus of the thalamus. It has one major afferent pathway, the anterior spinocerebellar tract.

2. The **middle cerebellar peduncle,** the largest cerebellar peduncle is connected to the brainstem at mid-pons, it contains the pontocerebellar fibers, which project to the neocerebellum (pontocerebellum).

3. The **inferior cerebellar peduncle,** connected to the caudal pons and rostral medulla, has three major afferent tracts: the posterior spinocerebellar tract, the cuneocerebellar tract, and the olivocerebellar tract from the contralateral inferior olivary nucleus.

C. Cerebellar Cortex, Neurons, and Fibers

1. The cerebellar cortex has three layers:

    a. The **molecular layer** is the most superficial, underlying the pia mater. It contains stellate cells, basket cells, and the dendritic arbor of the Purkinje cells.

    b. The **Purkinje cell layer** lies between the molecular and the granule cell layers.

    c. The **granule layer** is the deepest layer overlying the white matter. It contains granule cells, Golgi cells, and cerebellar glomeruli. A cerebellar glomerulus consists of a mossy fiber rosette, granule cell dendrites, and a Golgi cell axon.

2. Neurons and fibers of the cerebellum

    a. **Purkinje cells** convey the only output from the cerebellar cortex. They project inhibitory output (i.e., γ-aminobutyric acid [GABA]) to the cerebellar and vestibular nuclei. Purkinje cells are excited by parallel and climbing fibers and inhibited by GABA-ergic basket and stellate cells.

    b. **Granule cells** excite (by way of glutamate) Purkinje, basket, stellate, and Golgi cells through parallel fibers. They are inhibited by Golgi cells and excited by mossy fibers.

    c. **Parallel fibers** are the axons of granule cells. These fibers extend into the molecular layer.

    d. **Mossy fibers** are the afferent excitatory fibers of the spinocerebellar, pontocerebellar, and vestibulocerebellar tracts. They terminate as mossy fiber rosettes on granule cell dendrites. They excite granule cells to discharge through their parallel fibers.

    e. **Climbing fibers** are the afferent excitatory (by way of aspartate) fibers of the olivocerebellar tract. These fibers arise from the contralateral inferior olivary nucleus. They terminate on neurons of the cerebellar nuclei and dendrites of Purkinje cells.

 III   # The Deep Cerebellar Nuclei are found within the white matter and represent the output nuclei of the cerebellum. Functionally, the nuclei may be associated with more sophisticated function as one moves away from the midline (Table 1 and Figure 17-2).

A. Fastigial Nucleus—the most midline nucleus is associated with the paleocerebellum and deals with balance and equilibrium.

B. Interposed Nuclei (Globose and Emboliform)—associated with the archicerebellum deal with walking and arm movements.

C. Dentate Nucleus—the most lateral and the largest, is part of the neocerebellum and is associated with highly skilled movements, such as stacking a house of cards. Gives rise to dentatothalamic tract.

 IV   # The Major Cerebellar Circuit Influences ongoing motor activity. It consists of the following structures:

A. The **Purkinje cells of the cerebellar cortex** project to the deep cerebellar nuclei (e.g., dentate, interposed (emboliform and globose), and fastigial nuclei).

Table 17-1: Divisions of the Cerebellum

Anatomical	Phylogenetic	Functional	Deep Nucleus
Anterior lobe	Paleocerebellum	Spinal cerebellum	Interposed
	Primary fissure		
Posterior lobe	Neocerebellum	Cerebral cerebellum	Dentate
	Posterolateral fissure		
Flocculonodular lobe	Archicerebellum	Vestibular cerebellum	Fastigial

B. The **dentate nucleus** is the major effector nucleus of the cerebellum in humans. It gives rise to the dentatothalamic tract, which projects through the superior cerebellar peduncle to the contralateral ventral lateral nucleus of the thalamus. The decussation of the superior cerebellar peduncle is in the caudal midbrain tegmentum.

C. The **ventral lateral nucleus of the thalamus** receives the dentatothalamic tract. It projects to the primary motor cortex of the precentral gyrus (Brodmann area 4).

D. The **motor cortex (Brodmann area 4)** receives input from the ventral lateral nucleus of the thalamus. It projects as the corticopontine tract to the pontine nuclei.

E. The **pontine nuclei** receive input from the motor cortex. Axons project as the pontocerebellar tract to the contralateral cerebellar cortex, where they terminate as mossy fibers, thus completing the circuit.

 V Cerebellar Dysfunction includes the following triad:

A. Hypotonia is loss of the resistance normally offered by muscles to palpation or passive manipulation. It results in a floppy, loose-jointed, rag-doll appearance with pendular reflexes. The patient appears inebriated.

B. Dysequilibrium is loss of balance characterized by gait and trunk dystaxia.

C. Dyssynergia is loss of coordinated muscle activity. It includes **dysmetria, intention tremor,** failure to check movements, **nystagmus, dysdiadochokinesia,** and **dysrhythmokinesia. Cerebellar nystagmus** is coarse. It is more pronounced when the patient looks toward the side of the lesion.

 VI Cerebellar Syndromes and Tumors

A. Anterior Vermis Syndrome involves the lower limb region of the anterior lobe. It results from atrophy of the rostral vermis, most commonly caused by alcohol abuse. It causes gait, trunk, and lower limb dystaxia.

B. Posterior Vermis Syndrome involves the flocculonodular lobe. It is usually the result of brain tumors in children and is most commonly caused by medulloblastomas or ependymomas. It causes truncal dystaxia.

C. Hemispheric Syndrome usually involves one cerebellar hemisphere. It is often the result of a brain tumor (astrocytoma) or an abscess (secondary to otitis media or mastoiditis). It causes arm, leg, and gait dystaxia and ipsilateral cerebellar signs.

D. Cerebellar Tumors. In children, 70% of brain tumors are found infratentorially, in the posterior fossa. In adults, 70% of brain tumors are found in the supratentorial compartment.
   1. Astrocytomas constitute 30% of all brain tumors in children. They are most often found in the cerebellar hemisphere. After surgical removal of an astrocytoma, it is common for the child to survive for many years.
   2. Medulloblastomas are malignant and constitute 20% of all brain tumors in children. They are believed to originate from the superficial granule layer of the cerebellar cortex. They usually obstruct the passage of cerebrospinal fluid (CSF). As a result, hydrocephalus occurs.
   3. Ependymomas constitute 15% of all brain tumors in children. They occur most frequently in the fourth ventricle. They usually obstruct the passage of CSF and cause hydrocephalus.

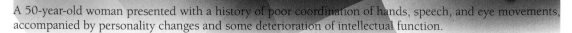

CASE 17-1

A 50-year-old woman presented with a history of poor coordination of hands, speech, and eye movements, accompanied by personality changes and some deterioration of intellectual function.

Relevant Physical Exam Findings

- Neurologic examination revealed marked cerebellar ataxia and spasticity of all extremities, held in a flexed posture. Babinski sign was negative. The sensory system appeared normal.

Relevant Lab Findings

- Laboratory results were unremarkable. A brain computed tomography scan showed generalized cerebral atrophy, most pronounced in the cerebellum.

Diagnosis

- Spinocerebellar ataxia is a genetic disease that is characterized by progressive loss of coordination of gait, with frequent involvement of hands, speech, and eye movements. At least 29 different gene mutations have been associated with the various forms of this disease.

CHAPTER 18

Cerebral Cortex

Objectives

1. Distinguish between the anatomical features of the neocortex and allocortex.
2. Summarize the cortical localization of the various functional areas of the brain, including sensory, motor, and higher association areas and their Brodmann areas.
3. How does the dominant hemisphere differ from the nondominant hemisphere?
4. Describe the anatomical basis of and functional deficits resulting from Gerstmann syndrome.
5. Describe and distinguish between the various types of apraxia, aphasia, and dysprosodies.

Introduction. The cerebral cortex, the thin, gray covering of both hemispheres of the brain, has two types: the neocortex (90%) and the allocortex (10%). Motor cortex is the thickest (4.5 mm); visual cortex is the thinnest (1.5 mm).

The Six-Layered Neocortex. Layers II and IV of the neocortex are mainly afferent (i.e., receiving). Layers V and VI are mainly efferent (i.e., sending) (Figure 18-1).

A. Layer I is the **molecular layer.**

B. Layer II is the **external granular** layer.

C. Layer III is the **external pyramidal** layer. It gives rise to association and commissural fibers and is the major source of corticocortical fibers.

D. Layer IV is the **internal granular** layer. It receives thalamocortical fibers from the thalamic nuclei of the ventral tier (i.e., ventral posterolateral and ventral posteromedial). In the visual cortex (area 17), layer IV receives input from the lateral geniculate body.

E. Layer V is the **internal pyramidal** layer. It gives rise to corticobulbar, corticospinal, and corticostriatal fibers. It contains the giant pyramidal cells of Betz, which are found only in the motor cortex (area 4).

F. Layer VI is the **multiform** layer. It is the **major source of corticothalamic fibers.** It gives rise to projection, commissural, and association fibers.

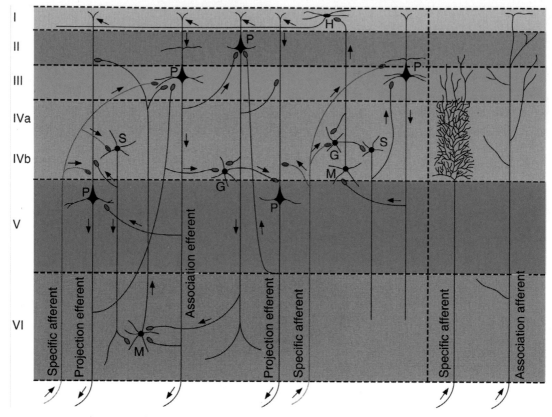

Figure 18-1 Neurocortical circuits. *G*, granule cell; *H*, horizontal cell; *M*, Martinotti cell; *P*, pyramidal cell; *S*, stellate cell. Loops show synaptic junctions. (Reprinted from Parent A. *Carpenter's Human Neuroanatomy*. 9th ed. Baltimore, MD: Williams & Wilkins; 1996:868, with permission.)

 III **Functional Areas** (Figure 18-2)

A. Frontal Lobe

1. The **motor cortex** (area 4) and **premotor cortex** (area 6). These two cortices are somatotopically organized (Figure 18-3). Destruction of these areas of the frontal lobe causes contralateral spastic paresis. Contralateral pronator drift is associated with frontal lobe lesions of the corticospinal tract.

2. **Frontal eye field** (area 8). Destruction causes deviation of the eyes to the ipsilateral side.

3. **Broca speech area** (areas 44 and 45). This is located in the posterior part of the inferior frontal gyrus in the dominant hemisphere (Figure 18-4). Destruction results in expressive, nonfluent aphasia (Broca aphasia). The patient understands both written and spoken language but cannot articulate speech or write normally. Broca aphasia is usually associated with contralateral facial and arm weakness because of the involvement of the motor strip.

4. **Prefrontal cortex** (areas 9 to 12 and 46 to 47). Destruction of the anterior two-thirds of the frontal lobe convexity results in deficits in concentration, orientation, abstracting ability, judgment, and problem-solving ability. Other frontal lobe deficits include loss of initiative, inappropriate behavior, release of sucking and grasping reflexes, gait apraxia, and sphincteric incontinence. Destruction of the orbital (frontal) lobe results in inappropriate social behavior (e.g., use of obscene language, urinating in public). Perseveration is associated with frontal lobe lesions.

B. Parietal Lobe

1. In the **sensory cortex** (areas 3, 1, and 2), which is somatotopically organized (see Figure 18-2), destruction results in contralateral hemihypesthesia and astereognosis.

A

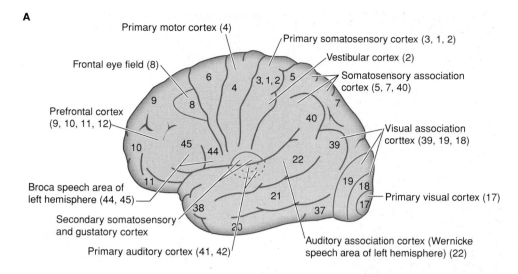

B

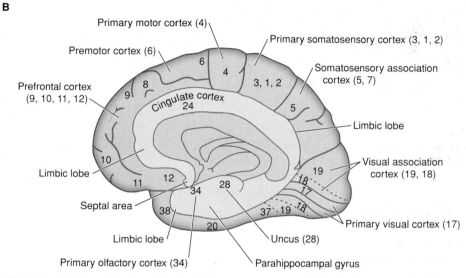

Figure 18-2 Motor and sensory areas of the cerebral cortex. **A.** Lateral convex surface of the hemisphere. **B.** Medial surface of the hemisphere. The numbers refer to the Brodmann brain map (Brodmann areas).

2. In the **superior parietal lobule** (areas 5 and 7), destruction results in contralateral astereognosis and sensory neglect.
3. In the **inferior parietal lobule** of the **dominant hemisphere,** damage results in Gerstmann syndrome, which includes the following deficits:
   a. **Right and left confusion**
   b. **Finger agnosia**
   c. **Dysgraphia and dyslexia**
   d. **Dyscalculia**
   e. **Contralateral hemianopia or lower quadrantanopia**
4. In the **inferior parietal lobule** of the **nondominant hemisphere,** destruction results in the following deficits:
   a. **Topographic memory loss**
   b. **Anosognosia**
   c. **Construction apraxia (Figure 18-5)**

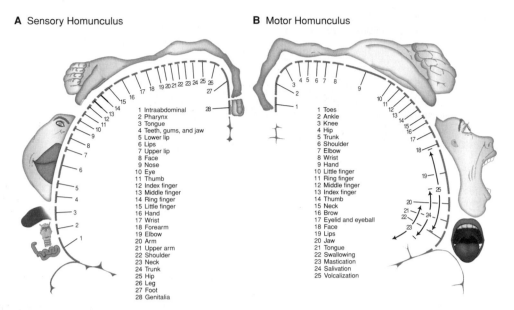

A Sensory Homunculus

B Motor Homunculus

1 Intraabdominal	1 Toes
2 Pharynx	2 Ankle
3 Tongue	3 Knee
4 Teeth, gums, and jaw	4 Hip
5 Lower lip	5 Trunk
6 Lips	6 Shoulder
7 Upper lip	7 Elbow
8 Face	8 Wrist
9 Nose	9 Hand
10 Eye	10 Little finger
11 Thumb	11 Ring finger
12 Index finger	12 Middle finger
13 Middle finger	13 Index finger
14 Ring finger	14 Thumb
15 Little finger	15 Neck
16 Hand	16 Brow
17 Wrist	17 Eyelid and eyeball
18 Forearm	18 Face
19 Elbow	19 Lips
20 Arm	20 Jaw
21 Upper arm	21 Tongue
22 Shoulder	22 Swallowing
23 Neck	23 Mastication
24 Trunk	24 Salivation
25 Hip	25 Volcalization
26 Leg	
27 Foot	
28 Genitalia	

Figure 18-3 The sensory and motor homunculi. **A.** Sensory representation in the postcentral gyrus. **B.** Motor representation in the precentral gyrus. (Reprinted from Penfield W, Rasmussen T. *The Cerebral Cortex of Man*. New York: Hafner; 1968:44, 57, with permission.)

    d. Dressing apraxia
    e. Contralateral sensory neglect
    f. Contralateral hemianopia or lower quadrantanopia

C. Temporal Lobe

    1. In the **primary auditory cortex** (areas 41 and 42), unilateral destruction results in slight loss of hearing. Bilateral loss results in cortical deafness.

    2. Wernicke speech area in the **dominant hemisphere** is found in the posterior part of the superior temporal gyrus (area 22). Destruction results in receptive, fluent aphasia (Wernicke aphasia),

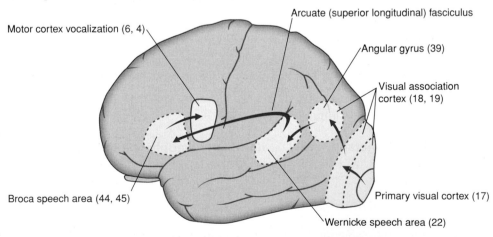

Figure 18-4 Cortical areas of the dominant hemisphere that play an important role in language production. The visual image of a word is projected from the visual cortex (Brodmann area 17) to the visual association cortices (Brodmann areas 18 and 19) and then to the angular gyrus (Brodmann area 39). Further processing occurs in Wernicke speech area (Brodmann area 22), where the auditory form of the word is recalled. Through the arcuate fasciculus, this information reaches Broca speech area (Brodmann areas 44 and 45), where motor speech programs control the vocalization mechanisms of the precentral gyrus. Lesions of Broca speech area, Wernicke speech area, or the arcuate fasciculus result in dysphasia.

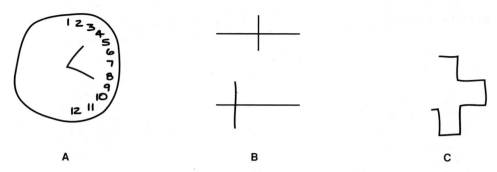

Figure 18-5 Testing for construction apraxia. **A.** The patient was asked to copy the face of a clock. **B.** The patient was asked to bisect a horizontal line. **C.** The patient was asked to copy a cross. These drawings show contralateral neglect. The responsible lesion is found in the nondominant (right) parietal lobe. A left hemianopia, by itself, does not result in contralateral neglect.

in which the patient cannot understand any form of language. Speech is spontaneous, fluent, and rapid, but makes little sense.

3. **Meyer loop** (see Chapter 14) consists of the visual radiations that project to the inferior bank of the calcarine sulcus. Interruption causes contralateral upper quadrantanopia ("pie in the sky").

4. **Olfactory bulb, tract,** and **primary cortex** (area 34) can see destruction that results in ipsilateral anosmia. An irritative lesion (psychomotor epilepsy) of the uncus results in olfactory and gustatory hallucinations.
   a. **Olfactory groove meningiomas** compress the olfactory tract and bulb, resulting in anosmia. See Foster Kennedy syndrome, Chapter 9.
   b. **Esthesioneuroblastomas** (olfactory neuroblastomas) arise from bipolar sensory cells of the olfactory mucosa; they can extend through the cribriform plate into the anterior cranial fossa. Presenting symptoms are similar to those of the Foster Kennedy syndrome.

5. In the **hippocampal cortex (archicortex),** bilateral lesions result in the inability to consolidate short-term memory into long-term memory. Earlier memories are retrievable.

6. In the **anterior temporal lobe,** including the **amygdaloid nucleus,** bilateral damage results in **Klüver–Bucy** syndrome, which consists of **psychic blindness** (visual agnosia), **hyperphagia,** docility, and **hypersexuality.**

7. In the **inferomedial occipitotemporal cortex,** bilateral lesions result in the inability to recognize once-familiar faces (prosopagnosia).

D. Occipital Lobe. Bilateral lesions cause cortical blindness. Unilateral lesions cause contralateral hemianopia or quadrantanopia.

 IV **Focal Destructive Hemispheric Lesions and Symptoms.** Figure 18-6A shows the symptoms of lesions in the dominant hemisphere. Figure 18-6B shows the symptoms of lesions in the nondominant hemisphere.

 V **Cerebral Dominance.** This dominance is determined by the **Wada test.** Sodium amobarbital (Amytal) is injected into the internal carotid artery. If the patient becomes aphasic, the anesthetic was administered to the dominant hemisphere.

A. The **dominant hemisphere** is usually the left hemisphere. It is responsible for **propositional language** (grammar, syntax, and semantics), speech, and calculation.

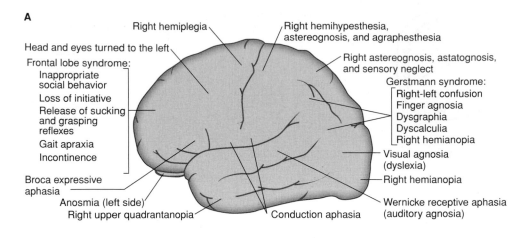

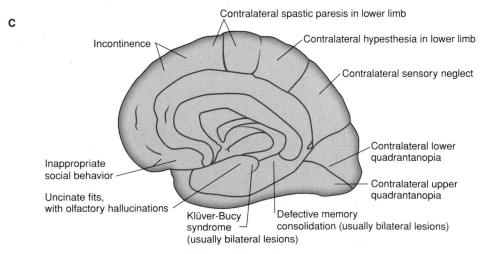

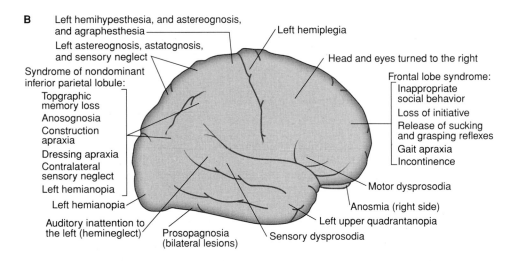

Figure 18-6 Focal destructive hemispheric lesions and the resulting symptoms. **A.** Lateral convex surface of the dominant left hemisphere. **B.** Lateral convex surface of the nondominant right hemisphere. **C.** Medial surface of the nondominant hemisphere.

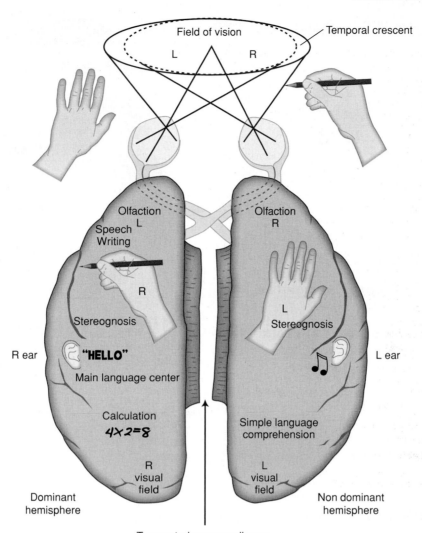

Figure 18-7 Functions of the split brain after transection of the corpus callosum. Tactile and visual perception is projected to the contralateral hemisphere, olfaction is perceived on the same side, and audition is perceived predominantly in the opposite hemisphere. The left (*L*) hemisphere is dominant for language. The right (*R*) hemisphere is dominant for spatial construction and nonverbal ideation. (Reprinted from Noback CR, Demarest RJ. *The Human Nervous System.* Malvern, PA: Lea & Febiger; 1991:416, with permission.)

B. The **nondominant hemisphere** is usually the right hemisphere. It is responsible for three-dimensional, or spatial, perception and nonverbal ideation. It also allows superior recognition of faces.

 VI Split Brain Syndrome (Figure 18-7). This syndrome is a disconnection syndrome that results from **transection** of the **corpus callosum.**

A. The **dominant hemisphere** is better at vocal naming.

B. The **nondominant, mute hemisphere** is better at pointing to a stimulus. A person cannot name objects that are presented to the nondominant visual cortex. A blindfolded person cannot name objects that are presented to the nondominant sensory cortex through touch.

C. Test (Figure 18-8). A subject views a composite picture of two half-faces (i.e., a chimeric, or hybrid, figure). The right side shows a man; the left side shows a woman. The picture is removed, and the subject is asked to describe what he saw. He may respond that he saw a man, but when asked to point to what he saw, he points to the woman.

D. In a patient who has **alexia** in the left visual field, the verbal symbols seen in the right visual cortex have no access to the language centers of the left hemisphere.

VII Other Lesions of the Corpus Callosum

A. Anterior Corpus Callosum Lesion may result in akinetic mutism or tactile anomia.

B. Posterior Corpus Callosum (Splenium) Lesion may result in alexia without agraphia.

C. Callosotomy has been successfully used to treat "drop attacks" (colloid cyst of third ventricle).

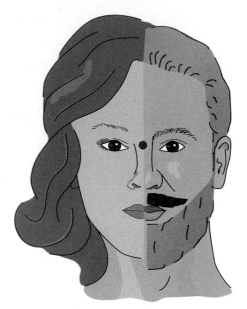

Figure 18-8 Chimeric (hybrid) figure of a face used to examine the hemispheric function of commissurotomized patients. The patient is instructed to fixate on the dot and is asked to describe what is seen. If the patient says that he or she sees the face of a man, the left hemisphere predominates in vocal tasks. If he or she is asked to point to the face and points to the woman, the right hemisphere predominates in pointing tasks.

VIII Brain and Spinal Cord Tumors (see Chapter 3)

IX Apraxia is the inability to perform motor activities in the presence of intact motor and sensory systems and normal comprehension.

A. Ideomotor Apraxia (Idiokenetic Apraxia)
1. The disorder results in loss of the ability to perform intransitive or imaginary gestures; the inability to perform complicated motor tasks (e.g., saluting, blowing a kiss, or making the "V" for victory sign)
2. The lesion is in Wernicke area.
3. **Bucco-facial or facial-oral apraxia** is a type of idiomotor apraxia; facial apraxia is the most common type of apraxia.

B. Ideational Apraxia (Ideatory Apraxia)
1. The inability to demonstrate the use of real objects (e.g., ask the patient to smoke a pipe, a multi-step complex sequence)
2. A misuse of objects owing to a disturbance of identification (agnosia)
3. The lesion in Wernicke area

C. Construction Apraxia (Figure 18-5), the inability to draw or construct a geometric figure (e.g., the face of a clock). If the patient draws only the right half of the clock, this condition is called *hemineglect,* and the lesion is located in the right inferior parietal lobule.

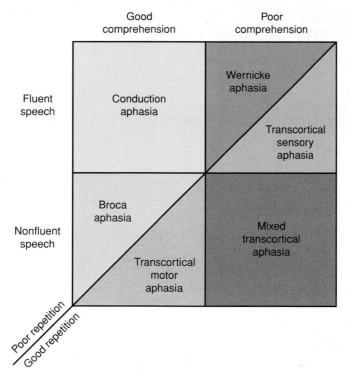

Figure 18-9 The "aphasia square" makes it easy to differentiate the six most common "national board" aphasias. Broca, conduction, and Wernicke aphasias are all characterized by poor repetition. (Adapted from Miller J, Fountain N. *Neurology Recall*. Baltimore, MD: Williams & Wilkins; 1997:35, with permission.)

D. Gait Apraxia, the inability to use the lower limbs properly. The patient has difficulty in lifting his feet from the floor, a frontal lobe sign seen with **normal-pressure hydrocephalus (gait apraxia, dementia, incontinence).**

 Aphasia is impaired or absent communication by speech, writing, or signs (i.e., loss of the capacity for spoken language). The lesions are located in the dominant hemisphere. Associate the following symptoms and lesion sites with the appropriate aphasia (Figure 18-9).

A. Broca (Motor) Aphasia
1. Lesion in frontal lobe, in the inferior frontal gyrus (areas 44 and 45)
2. Good comprehension
3. Effortful speech
4. Dysarthric speech
5. Telegraphic speech
6. Nonfluent speech
7. Poor repetition
8. Contralateral lower facial and upper limb weakness

B. Wernicke (Sensory) Aphasia
1. Lesion in posterior temporal lobe, in the superior temporal gyrus (area 22)
2. Poor comprehension
3. Fluent speech
4. Poor repetition

5. Quadrantanopia
6. **Paraphasic errors**
   a. **Non sequiturs** (Latin, "does not follow"): statements irrelevant to the question asked
   b. **Neologisms:** words with no meaning
   c. **Driveling speech**

C. Conduction Aphasia

1. **Transection of the arcuate fasciculus;** the arcuate fasciculus interconnects Brodmann speech area with Wernicke speech area.
2. Poor repetition
3. Good comprehension
4. Fluent speech

D. Transcortical Motor Aphasia

1. Poor comprehension
2. Good repetition
3. Nonfluent speech

E. Transcortical Mixed Aphasia

1. Poor comprehension
2. Good repetition
3. Nonfluent speech

F. Transcortical Sensory Aphasia

1. Poor comprehension
2. Good repetition
3. Fluent speech

G. Global Aphasia.
Resulting from a lesion of the perisylvian area, which contains Broca and Wernicke areas, global aphasia combines all of the symptoms of Broca and Wernicke aphasias.

H. Thalamic Aphasia.
A dominant thalamic syndrome, thalamic aphasia closely resembles a thought disorder of patients with schizophrenia and chronic drug-induced psychosis. Symptoms include fluent paraphasic speech with normal comprehension and repetition.

I. Basal Nuclei.
Diseases of the basal nuclei may cause aphasia. Lesions of the anterior basal nuclei result in nonfluent aphasia. Lesions of the posterior basal nuclei result in fluent aphasia.

J. Watershed Infarcts.
Such infarcts are areas of infarction in the boundary zones of the anterior, middle, and posterior cerebral arteries. These areas are vulnerable to hypoperfusion and thus may separate Broca and Wernicke speech areas from the surrounding cortex. These infarcts cause the motor, mixed, and sensory transcortical aphasias.

XI   **Dysprosodies** are nondominant hemispheric language deficits that serve propositional language. Emotionality, inflection, melody, emphasis, and gesturing are affected.

A. Expressive Dysprosody
results from a lesion that corresponds to Broca area but is located in the nondominant hemisphere. Patients cannot express emotion or inflection in their speech.

B. Receptive Dysprosody
results from a lesion that corresponds to Wernicke area but is located in the nondominant hemisphere. Patients cannot comprehend the emotionality or inflection in the speech they hear.

CASE 18-1

A 50-year-old woman was referred to neurology with a year-long history of poor memory and speech difficulties. She noted an inability to remember the names of common household objects and complained of forgetting her friends' names. She complained of becoming indecisive, such that she had significant difficulty in making straightforward decisions and in processing new information.

Physical Exam Findings

- On testing higher cortical function, her speech was somewhat rambling and hesitant, with word-finding difficulty. The neurologic examination was otherwise normal.

Relevant Lab Findings

- Single-photon emission computed tomography cerebral perfusion disclosed markedly reduced perfusion in the left temporal and parietal lobes and the right posterior parietal regions.

Diagnosis

- Aphasia is a language disorder resulting from damage to brain regions responsible for language (left hemisphere). Onset may occur either suddenly, owing to trauma, or slowly, as in the case of a brain tumor. Aphasia impairs expression and understanding of language and reading and writing.

CHAPTER 19

Cross-Sectional Anatomy of the Brain

Objective

1. Identify the major structures of the brain from the three orthogonal planes, including sagittal, coronal, and axial sections.

 Introduction. Thick, stained brain slices in this chapter are accompanied by corresponding magnetic resonance imaging scans. Together they represent a **mini-atlas** of brain slices in the three orthogonal planes (i.e., midsagittal, coronal, and axial). An insert on each figure shows the level of the slice. The most commonly tested structures are labeled.

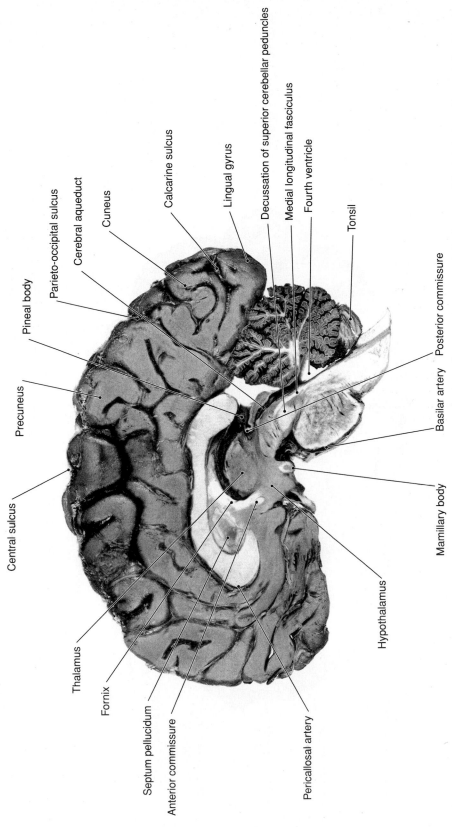

Figure 19-1 Midsagittal section of the brain with meninges and blood vessels intact. Arachnoid granulations are seen along the crest of the hemisphere. The posterior commissure, decussation of the superior cerebellar peduncles, and medial longitudinal fasciculus are well demonstrated. (Modified from Roberts M, Hanaway J, Morest DK. *Atlas of the Human Brain in Section*. 2nd ed. Philadelphia, PA: Lea & Febiger; 1987:85.)

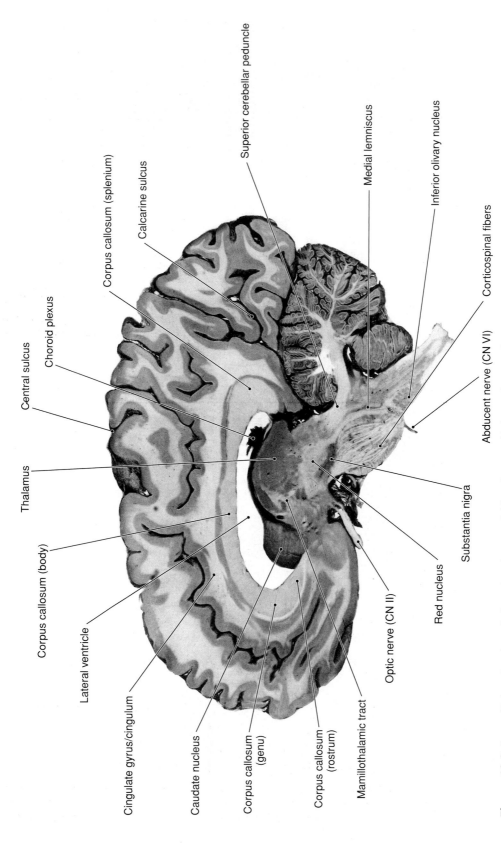

Figure 19-2 Parasagittal section through the red nucleus, medial lemniscus, and inferior olivary nucleus. The corticospinal fibers can be traced from the crus cerebri to the spinal cord. The abducent nerve (CN VI) is seen exiting from the junction of the pons and medulla. (Modified from Roberts M, Hanaway J, Morest DK. *Atlas of the Human Brain in Section.* 2nd ed. Philadelphia, PA: Lea & Febiger; 1987:81.)

Superior cerebellar peduncle

Corpus callosum (splenium)

Calcarine sulcus

Choroid plexus

Central sulcus

Thalamus

Corpus callosum (body)

Lateral ventricle

Cingulate gyrus/cingulum

Caudate nucleus

Corpus callosum (genu)

Corpus callosum (rostrum)

Mamillothalamic tract

Optic nerve (CN II)

Red nucleus

Substantia nigra

Abducent nerve (CN VI)

Corticospinal fibers

Inferior olivary nucleus

Medial lemniscus

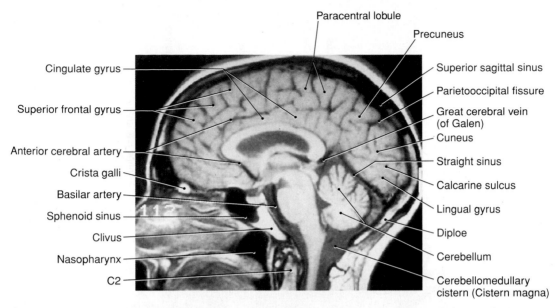

Figure 19-3 Midsagittal magnetic resonance imaging section through the brain and brain stem showing the important structures surrounding the third and fourth ventricles. This is a T1-weighted image. The gray matter appears gray (hypointense), whereas the white matter appears white (hyperintense).

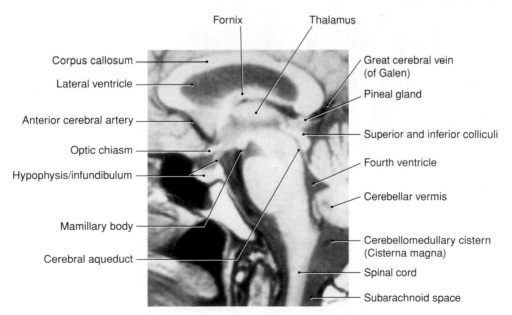

Figure 19-4 Midsagittal magnetic resonance imaging section through the brain stem and diencephalon. Note the cerebrospinal fluid tract: lateral ventricle, cerebral aqueduct, fourth ventricle, cerebellomedullary cistern (cisterna magna), and spinal subarachnoid space. Note also the relation between the optic chiasm, infundibulum, and hypophysis (pituitary gland).

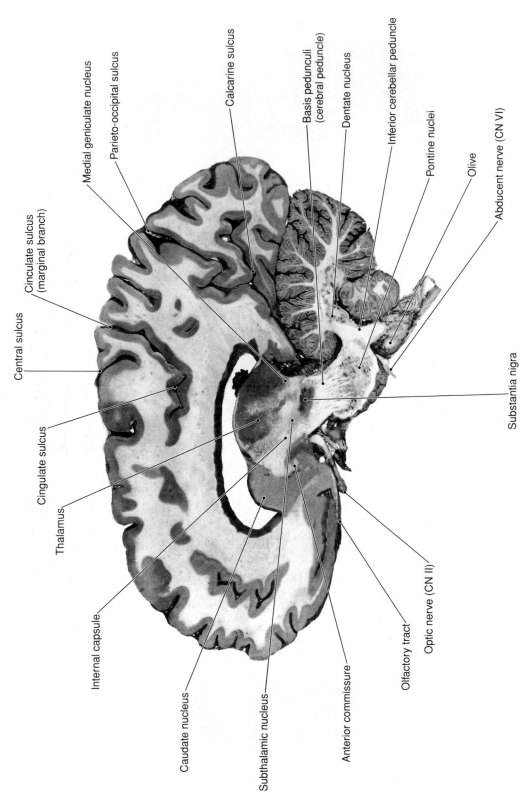

Figure 19-5 Parasagittal section through the caudate nucleus, subthalamic nucleus, substantia nigra, and dentate nucleus. (Modified from Roberts M, Hanaway J, Morest DK. *Atlas of the Human Brain in Section.* 2nd ed. Philadelphia, PA: Lea & Febiger; 1987:79.)

Central sulcus

Cinculate sulcus (marginal branch)

Medial geniculate nucleus

Parieto-occipital sulcus

Calcarine sulcus

Basis pedunculi (cerebral peduncle)

Dentate nucleus

Inferior cerebellar peduncle

Pontine nuclei

Olive

Abducent nerve (CN VI)

Cingulate sulcus

Thalamus

Internal capsule

Caudate nucleus

Subthalamic nucleus

Anterior commissure

Olfactory tract

Optic nerve (CN II)

Substantia nigra

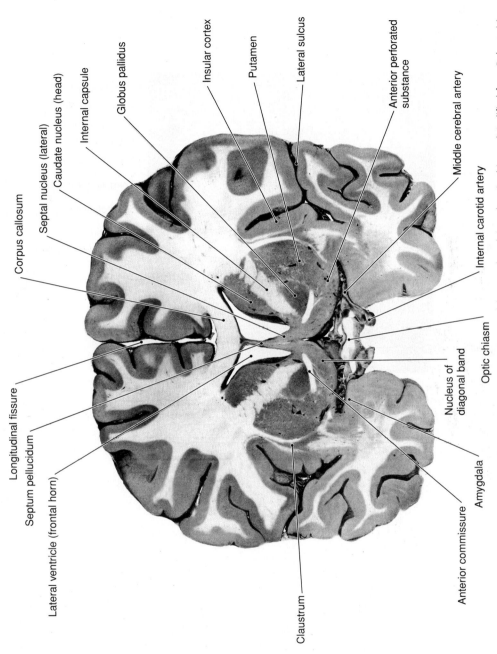

Figure 19-6 Coronal section through the anterior commissure, amygdala, septal nuclei, and optic chiasm. (Modified from Roberts M, Hanaway J, Morest DK. *Atlas of the Human Brain in Section.* 2nd ed. Philadelphia, PA: Lea & Febiger; 1987:9.)

Longitudinal fissure

Septum pellucidum

Lateral ventricle (frontal horn)

Corpus callosum

Septal nucleus (lateral)

Caudate nucleus (head)

Internal capsule

Globus pallidus

Insular cortex

Putamen

Lateral sulcus

Anterior perforated substance

Middle cerebral artery

Internal carotid artery

Optic chiasm

Nucleus of diagonal band

Amygdala

Anterior commissure

Claustrum

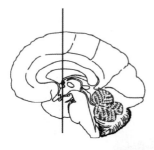

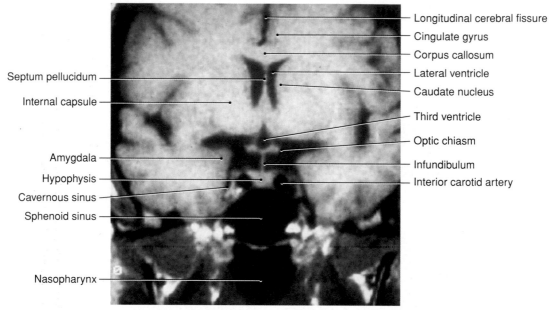

Septum pellucidum —

Internal capsule —

Amygdala —

Hypophysis —

Cavernous sinus —

Sphenoid sinus —

Nasopharynx —

— Longitudinal cerebral fissure

— Cingulate gyrus

— Corpus callosum

— Lateral ventricle

— Caudate nucleus

— Third ventricle

— Optic chiasm

— Infundibulum

— Interior carotid artery

Figure 19-7 Coronal magnetic resonance imaging section through the amygdala, optic chiasm, infundibulum, and internal capsule. The cavernous sinus encircles the sella turcica and contains the following structures: cranial nerves (CN) III, IV, VI, V_1, and V_2; postganglionic sympathetic fibers; and the internal carotid artery. This is a T1-weighted image.

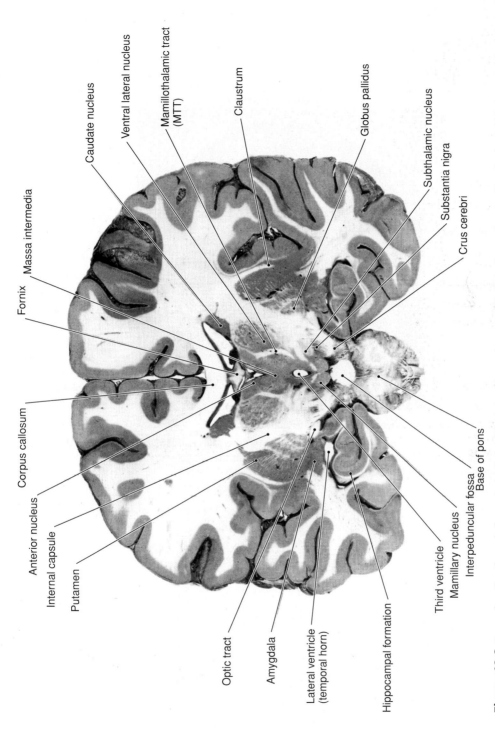

Figure 19-8 Coronal section through the posterior limb of the internal capsule, mammillothalamic tract, mammillary body, and hippocampal formation. The optic tracts are visible bilaterally. (Modified from Roberts M, Hanaway J, Morest DK. *Atlas of the Human Brain in Section.* 2nd ed. Philadelphia, PA: Lea & Febiger; 1987:19.)

Massa intermedia

Fornix

Corpus callosum

Anterior nucleus

Internal capsule

Putamen

Caudate nucleus

Ventral lateral nucleus

Mamillothalamic tract (MTT)

Claustrum

Globus pallidus

Subthalamic nucleus

Substantia nigra

Crus cerebri

Base of pons

Interpeduncular fossa

Mamillary nucleus

Third ventricle

Hippocampal formation

Lateral ventricle (temporal horn)

Amygdala

Optic tract

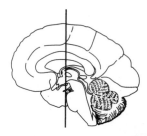

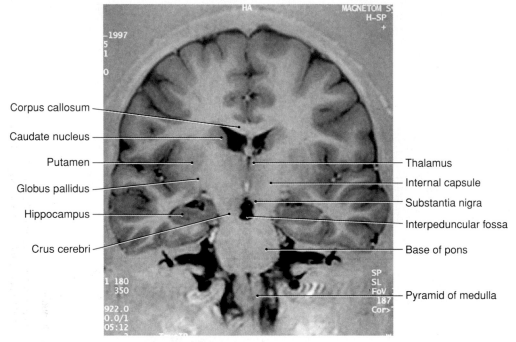

Corpus callosum

Caudate nucleus

Putamen

Globus pallidus

Hippocampus

Crus cerebri

Thalamus

Internal capsule

Substantia nigra

Interpeduncular fossa

Base of pons

Pyramid of medulla

Figure 19-9 Coronal magnetic resonance imaging section of the brain and brainstem at the level of the thalamus, and hippocampal formation. Note that the posterior limb of the internal capsule lies between the thalamus and the lentiform nucleus (putamen and globus pallidus). This is a T1-weighted postcontrast image.

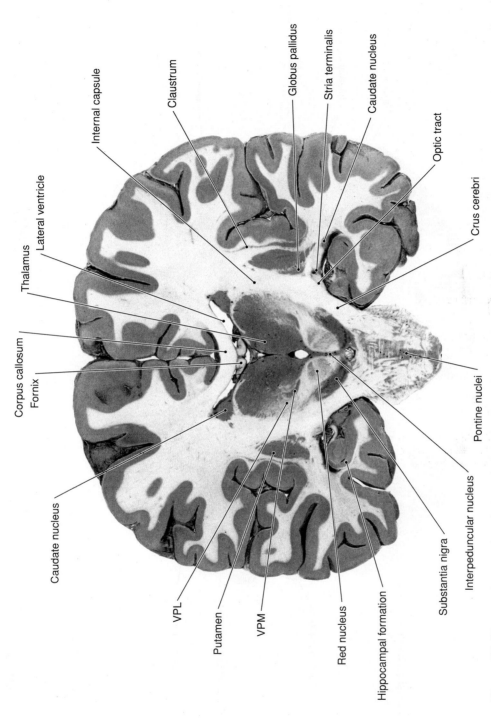

Figure 19-10 Coronal section through the thalamus, ventral posteromedial nucleus (*VPM*) and the ventral posterolateral nucleus (*VPL*), posterior limb of the internal capsule, substantia nigra, and red nucleus. (Modified from Roberts M, Hanaway J, Morest DK. *Atlas of the Human Brain in Section.* 2nd ed. Philadelphia, PA: Lea & Febiger; 1987:23.)

Internal capsule

Claustrum

Globus pallidus

Stria terminalis

Caudate nucleus

Optic tract

Crus cerebri

Lateral ventricle

Thalamus

Corpus callosum

Fornix

Caudate nucleus

VPL

Putamen

VPM

Red nucleus

Hippocampal formation

Substantia nigra

Interpeduncular nucleus

Pontine nuclei

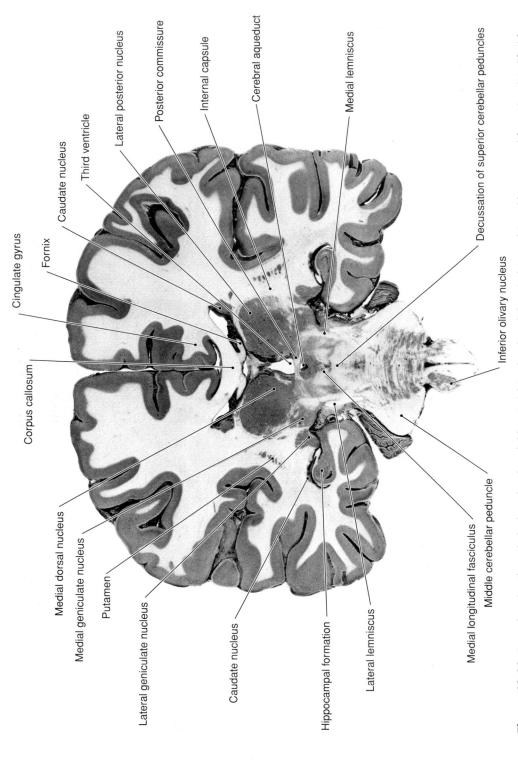

Figure 19-11 Coronal section through the lateral and medial lemnisci, lateral and medial geniculate nuclei, and hippocampal formation. (Modified from Roberts M, Hanaway J, Morest DK. *Atlas of the Human Brain in Section*. 2nd ed. Philadelphia, PA: Lea & Febiger; 1987:25.)

Cingulate gyrus

Fornix

Caudate nucleus

Third ventricle

Lateral posterior nucleus

Posterior commissure

Internal capsule

Cerebral aqueduct

Medial lemniscus

Decussation of superior cerebellar peduncles

Inferior olivary nucleus

Middle cerebellar peduncle

Medial longitudinal fasciculus

Lateral lemniscus

Hippocampal formation

Caudate nucleus

Lateral geniculate nucleus

Putamen

Medial geniculate nucleus

Medial dorsal nucleus

Corpus callosum

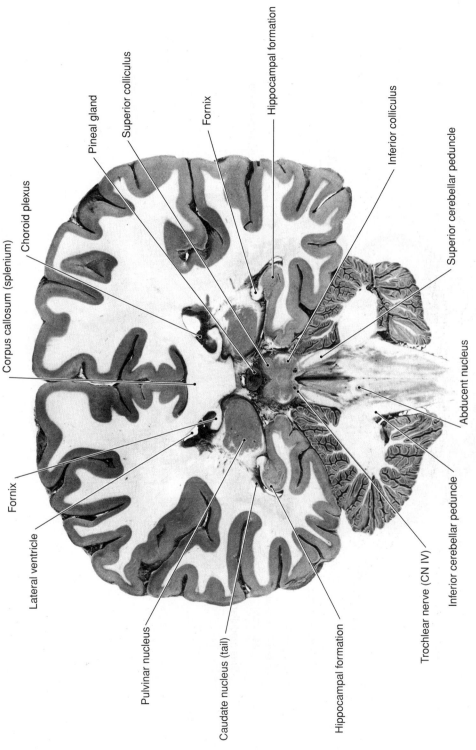

Figure 19-12 Coronal section through the pulvinar, pineal gland (epiphysis), superior and inferior colliculi, and trochlear nerve (CN IV). (Modified from Roberts M, Hanaway J, Morest DK. *Atlas of the Human Brain in Section.* 2nd ed. Philadelphia, PA: Lea & Febiger; 1987:29.)

Corpus callosum (splenium)

Choroid plexus

Pineal gland

Superior colliculus

Fornix

Hippocampal formation

Inferior colliculus

Superior cerebellar peduncle

Abducent nucleus

Fornix

Lateral ventricle

Pulvinar nucleus

Caudate nucleus (tail)

Hippocampal formation

Trochlear nerve (CN IV)

Inferior cerebellar peduncle

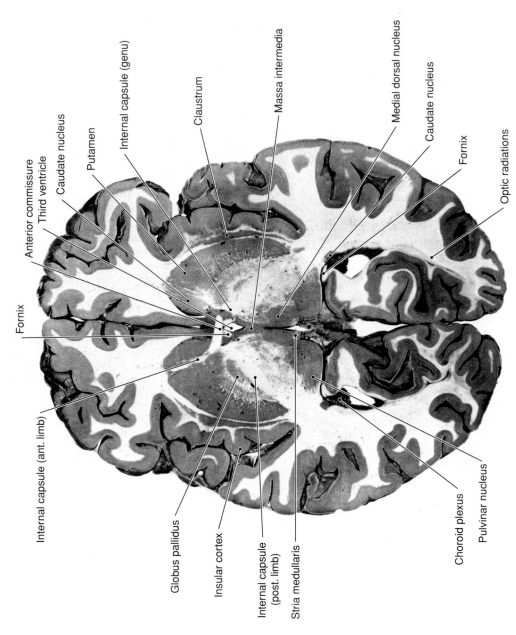

Figure 19-13 Axial section through the internal capsule, anterior commissure, and pulvinar nucleus. (Modified from Roberts M, Hanaway J, Morest DK. *Atlas of the Human Brain in Section.* 2nd ed. Philadelphia, PA: Lea & Febiger; 1987:51.)

Fornix

Anterior commissure

Third ventricle

Caudate nucleus

Putamen

Internal capsule (genu)

Claustrum

Massa intermedia

Medial dorsal nucleus

Caudate nucleus

Fornix

Optic radiations

Internal capsule (ant. limb)

Globus pallidus

Insular cortex

Internal capsule (post. limb)

Stria medullaris

Choroid plexus

Pulvinar nucleus

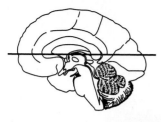

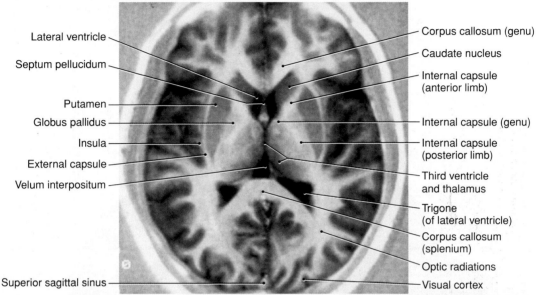

Lateral ventricle
Septum pellucidum
Putamen
Globus pallidus
Insula
External capsule
Velum interpositum
Superior sagittal sinus

Corpus callosum (genu)
Caudate nucleus
Internal capsule (anterior limb)
Internal capsule (genu)
Internal capsule (posterior limb)
Third ventricle and thalamus
Trigone (of lateral ventricle)
Corpus callosum (splenium)
Optic radiations
Visual cortex

Figure 19-14 Axial magnetic resonance imaging section at the level of the internal capsule and basal nuclei (ganglia). Note that the caudate nucleus bulges into the frontal horn of the lateral ventricle. In Huntington's disease, there is a massive loss of γ-aminobutyric acid (GABA)-ergic neurons in the caudate nucleus that results in hydrocephalus ex vacuo. A lesion of the genu of the internal capsule results in a contralateral weak lower face with sparing of the upper face. This is a T1-weighted image.

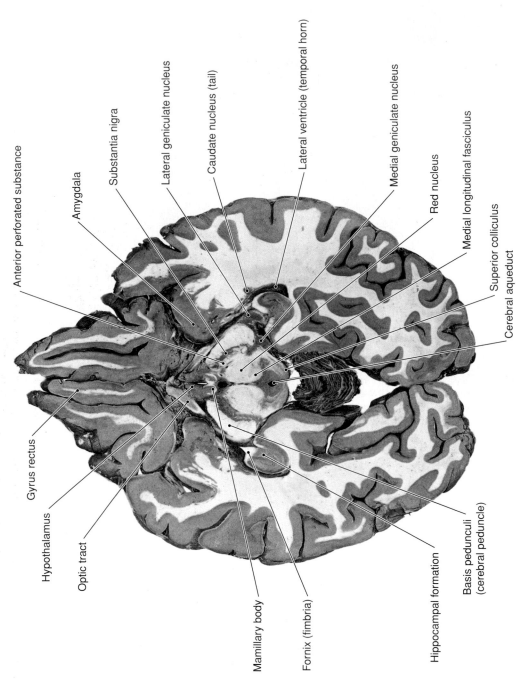

Figure 19-15 Axial section through the mammillary nuclei and the superior colliculi. (Modified from Roberts M, Hanaway J, Morest DK. *Atlas of the Human Brain in Section*. 2nd ed. Philadelphia, PA: Lea & Febiger; 1987:57.)

Anterior perforated substance

Amygdala

Substantia nigra

Lateral geniculate nucleus

Caudate nucleus (tail)

Lateral ventricle (temporal horn)

Medial geniculate nucleus

Red nucleus

Medial longitudinal fasciculus

Superior colliculus

Cerebral aqueduct

Gyrus rectus

Hypothalamus

Optic tract

Mamillary body

Fornix (fimbria)

Hippocampal formation

Basis pedunculi (cerebral peduncle)

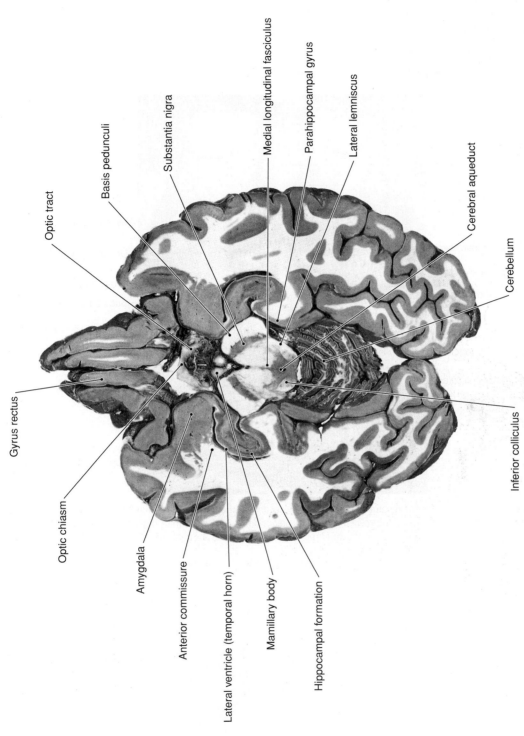

Figure 19-16 Axial section through the mammillary nuclei, optic chiasm, and inferior colliculi. (Modified from Roberts M, Hanaway J, Morest DK. *Atlas of the Human Brain in Section*. 2nd ed. Philadelphia, PA: Lea & Febiger; 1987:59.)

Optic tract

Basis pedunculi

Substantia nigra

Medial longitudinal fasciculus

Parahippocampal gyrus

Lateral lemniscus

Cerebral aqueduct

Cerebellum

Gyrus rectus

Optic chiasm

Amygdala

Anterior commissure

Lateral ventricle (temporal horn)

Mamillary body

Hippocampal formation

Inferior colliculus

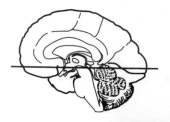

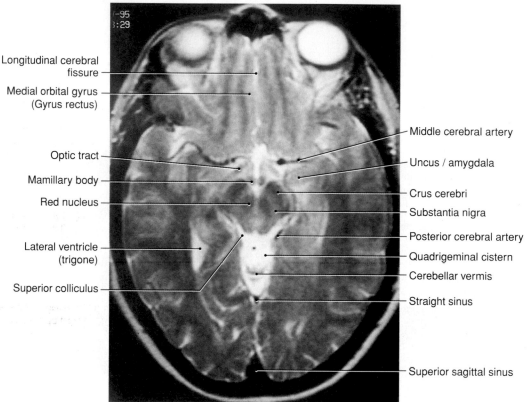

Longitudinal cerebral fissure

Medial orbital gyrus (Gyrus rectus)

Optic tract

Mamillary body

Red nucleus

Lateral ventricle (trigone)

Superior colliculus

Middle cerebral artery

Uncus / amygdala

Crus cerebri

Substantia nigra

Posterior cerebral artery

Quadrigeminal cistern

Cerebellar vermis

Straight sinus

Superior sagittal sinus

Figure 19-17 Axial magnetic resonance imaging (MRI) section at the level of the midbrain and mammillary bodies. Because of the high iron content, the red nuclei, mammillary bodies, and substantia nigra show a reduced MRI signal in T2-weighted images. Flowing blood in the cerebral vessels stands out as a signal void. Cerebrospinal fluid produces a strong signal in the ventricles and cisterns.

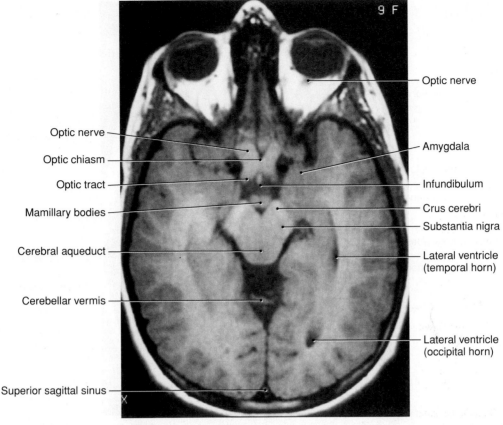

Figure 19-18 Axial magnetic resonance imaging section at the level of the optic chiasm, mammillary bodies, and midbrain. This patient has neurofibromatosis type 1 and an optic nerve glioma. Note the size of the right optic nerve. The infundibulum is postfixed. This is a T1-weighted image.

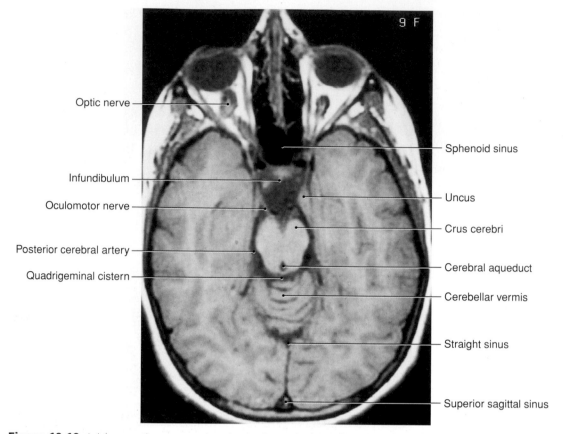

Figure 19-19 Axial magnetic resonance imaging section at the level of the uncal incisure, oculomotor nerve.

CHAPTER 20

Neurotransmitters

Objectives

1. List the major neurotransmitters.
2. Describe acetylcholine's targets and its role in Alzheimer disease.
3. Describe the catecholamines and serotonin. Give examples of each, their role, and location(s).
4. Describe and give examples of opioids. Compare and contrast opioids and nonopioid peptides.
5. Describe the amino acid neurotransmitters, give examples of each.
6. Describe the role of neurotransmitters in Parkinson disease, Huntington chorea, Myasthenia gravis, and Lambert–Eaton myasthenic syndrome.

Major Neurotransmitters

A. Acetylcholine is the major transmitter of the peripheral nervous system, neuromuscular junction, parasympathetic nervous system, and preganglionic sympathetic fibers. Acetylcholine is found in the neurons of the somatic and visceral motor nuclei in the brain stem and spinal cord. The largest concentration of acetylcholine in the CNS is found in the **basal nucleus of Meynert,** which degenerates in **Alzheimer disease** (Figure 20-1).

B. Catecholamines. Figure 20-2 shows the biosynthetic pathway for catecholamines. Epinephrine plays an insignificant role as a CNS neurotransmitter; it is found only in small neuronal clusters in the medulla. In the body, epinephrine is found primarily in the adrenal medulla.

Acetylcholine (ACh)

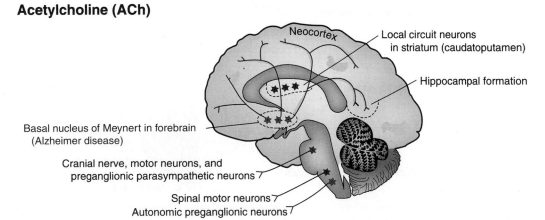

Figure 20-1 Distribution of acetylcholine-containing neurons and their axonal projections. The basal nucleus of Meynert projects to the entire cortex. This nucleus degenerates in patients with Alzheimer disease. Striatal acetylcholine local circuit neurons degenerate in patients with Huntington disease.

1. **Dopamine (Figure 20-3)** is depleted in patients with Parkinson disease and increased in patients with schizophrenia. Dopamine is found in the arcuate nucleus of the hypothalamus. It is the **prolactin-inhibiting factor.** Its two major receptors are D_1 and D_2.
   a. **D_1 receptors** are postsynaptic. They activate adenylate cyclase and are excitatory.
   b. **D_2 receptors** are both postsynaptic and presynaptic. They inhibit adenylate cyclase and are inhibitory. Antipsychotic drugs block D_2 receptors.

2. **Norepinephrine (Figure 20-4)** is the neurotransmitter of most postganglionic sympathetic neurons—exceptions include sweat glands and some blood vessels that receive acetylcholine. Antidepressant drugs enhance norepinephrine transmission.
   a. Norepinephrine plays a role in **anxiety. Panic attacks** are believed to result from paroxysmal discharges from the **locus ceruleus,** where norepinephrin-

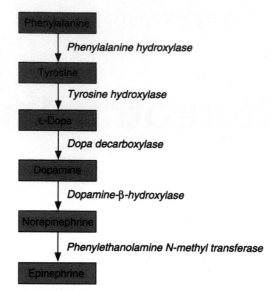

Figure 20-2 Synthesis of catecholamines from phenylalanine. Epinephrine, which is derived from norepinephrine, is found primarily in the adrenal medulla.

ergic neurons are found in the highest concentration. Most postsynaptic receptors of the locus ceruleus pathway are β_1 or β_2 receptors that activate adenylate cyclase and are excitatory.

3. The **catecholamine hypothesis of mood disorders** indicates that reduced norepinephrine and dopamine in the brain is related to depression and that increased norepinephrine activity is related to mania.

C. Serotonin (5-hydroxytryptamine [5-HT])

C. Serotonin (5-hydroxytryptamine [5-HT]) is an indolamine (Figure 20-5). Serotonin-containing neurons are found only in the **raphe nuclei** of the brain stem.

1. The **permissive hypothesis** states that the control of emotional behavior results from a balance between norepinephrine and serotonin.

Dopamine

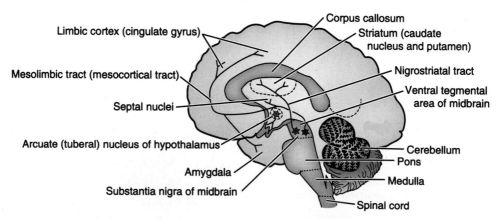

Figure 20-3 Distribution of dopamine-containing neurons and their projections. Two major ascending dopamine pathways arise in the midbrain: the nigrostriatal tract from the substantia nigra and the mesolimbic tract from the ventral tegmental area. In patients with Parkinson disease, loss of dopaminergic neurons occurs in the substantia nigra and the ventral tegmental area. Dopaminergic neurons from the arcuate nucleus of the hypothalamus project to the portal vessels of the infundibulum. Dopaminergic neurons inhibit prolactin.

Norepinephrine (NE)

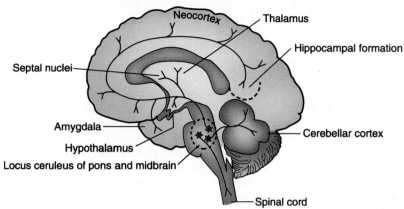

Figure 20-4 Distribution of norepinephrine-containing neurons and their projections. The locus ceruleus (located in the pons and midbrain) is the chief source of noradrenergic fibers. The locus ceruleus projects to all parts of the central nervous system.

   2. Certain **antidepressants** increase 5-HT availability by reducing its reuptake. 5-HT agonists that bind 5-HT_{1A} and those that block 5-HT_2 have antidepressant properties. Fluoxetine is a selective serotonin reuptake inhibitor.

D. Opioid Peptides (Endogenous Opiates) are short amino acid sequences that bind to opioid receptors—G protein–coupled receptors, exogenous opiates, such as morphine also activate opioid receptors.
   1. Endorphins are inhibitory neuropeptides. β-Endorphin is the major endorphin in the brain. They inhibit pain transmission and produce feelings of euphoria.

Serotonin (5-HT)

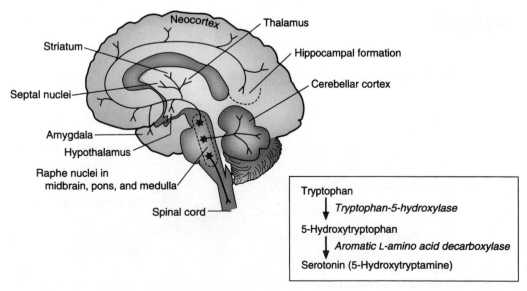

Figure 20-5 Distribution of 5-hydroxytryptamine (serotonin)–containing neurons and their projections. Serotonin-containing neurons are found in the nuclei of the raphe. They project widely to the forebrain, cerebellum, and spinal cord. The *inset* shows the synthetic pathway of serotonin.

2. **Enkephalins** are the most widely distributed and abundant opiate peptides. They are found in the highest concentration in the globus pallidus. They play a role in pain suppression.
3. **Dynorphins** are opioid peptides that are synthesized widely throughout the CNS. They moderate pain response.

E. Nonopioid Neuropeptides

1. **Substance P** is a neuropeptide that functions in pain modulation and in signaling the intensity of noxious stimuli, more recently its role in psychologic stress has been described. It plays a role in **movement disorders**—substance P levels are **reduced** in patients with **Huntington disease.**
2. **Somatostatin (somatotropin-release–inhibiting factor).** Somatostatinergic neurons from the anterior hypothalamus project their axons to the median eminence, where somatostatin enters the hypophyseal portal system and **regulates the release of growth hormone** and **thyroid-stimulating hormone.** The concentration of somatostatin in the neocortex and hippocampus is significantly **reduced** in patients with **Alzheimer disease.** Striatal somatostatin levels are **increased** in patients with **Huntington disease.**

F. Amino Acid Transmitters

1. **Inhibitory amino acid transmitters**
   a. **GABA (Figure 20-6)** is the major inhibitory neurotransmitter of the brain. Purkinje, stellate, basket, and Golgi cells of the cerebellar cortex are GABA-ergic.
      i. *GABA-ergic striatal neurons* project to the globus pallidus and substantia nigra.
      ii. *GABA-ergic pallidal neurons* project to the thalamus.
      iii. *GABA-ergic nigral neurons* project to the thalamus.
      iv. *GABA receptors* (GABA-A and GABA-B) are intimately associated with benzodiazepine-binding sites. Benzodiazepines enhance GABA activity.
   b. **Glycine** is a major inhibitory neurotransmitter of the spinal cord, brainstem, and retina. It is used by the Renshaw cells of the spinal cord.
2. **Excitatory amino acid transmitters**
   a. **Glutamate (Figure 20-7)** is the **major excitatory neurotransmitter of the CNS.** Neocortical glutamatergic neurons project to the striatum, subthalamic nucleus, and thalamus.
      i. Glutamate is the transmitter of the cerebellar granule cells, of nonnociceptive, large, primary afferent fibers that enter the spinal cord and brainstem, and of the corticonuclear and corticospinal tracts.

γ-Aminobutyric acid (GABA)

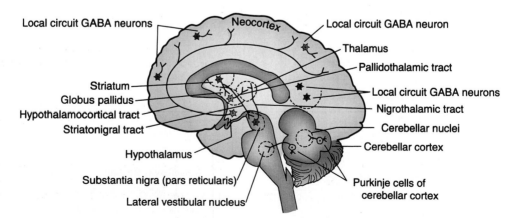

Figure 20-6 Distribution of γ-aminobutyric acid (*GABA*)-containing neurons and their projections. GABA-ergic neurons are the major inhibitory cells of the central nervous system. GABA local circuit neurons are found in the neocortex, hippocampal formation, and cerebellar cortex (Purkinje cells). Striatal GABA-ergic neurons project to the thalamus and subthalamic nucleus (not shown).

Glutamate

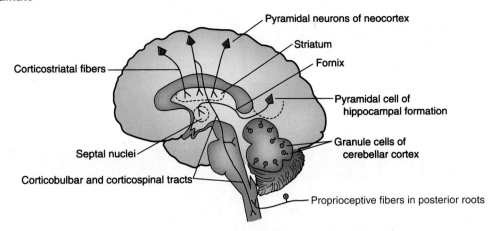

Figure 20-7 Distribution of glutamate-containing neurons and their projections. Glutamate is the major excitatory transmitter of the central nervous system. Cortical glutamatergic neurons project to the striatum. Hippocampal and subicular glutamatergic neurons project through the fornix to the septal area and hypothalamus. The granule cells of the cerebellum are glutamatergic.

> *ii.* Glutamate binding activates AMPA and NMDA receptors postsynaptically.
>
> *iii.* More recently, glutamate's role in long-term potentiation, as related to learning and memory, has been described.
>
> *iv. Glutamate excitotoxicity.* Glutamate is released in the striatum and binds to receptors on striatal neurons, resulting in an action potential. In Huntington disease, it is bound to the NMDA receptor, resulting in an influx of calcium ions and subsequent cell death. This cascade of events most likely occurs in cerebrovascular accidents (stroke).
>
> **b. Aspartate** is the excitatory neurotransmitter of the climbing fibers of the cerebellum. Neurons giving rise to climbing fibers are found in the inferior olivary nucleus.
>
> **3. Nitric oxide** is produced when nitric oxide synthase converts arginine to citrulline.
>
> **a.** It is a relatively ubiquitous neurotransmitter, located in the olfactory system, striatum, neocortex, hippocampal formation, supraoptic nucleus of the hypothalamus, and cerebellum.
>
> **b.** Nitric oxide is responsible for smooth-muscle relaxation of the corpus cavernosum and thus penile erection.

II Functional and Clinical Considerations

A. Parkinson Disease results from degeneration of the dopaminergic neurons in the pars compacta of the substantia nigra. It causes a reduction of dopamine in the striatum and substantia nigra (see Chapter 16, III.A).

B. Huntington Disease (Chorea) is a genetic disorder that results from a loss of acetylcholine- and GABA-containing neurons in the striatum. It is characterized by atrophy of the caudate and putamen, chorea, cognitive impairment and psychiatric disorders.

C. Alzheimer Disease results, in part, from the degeneration of cortical neurons and cholinergic neurons in the **basal nucleus of Meynert.** It is characterized by the presence of **neurofibrillary tangles, senile (neuritic) plaques, amyloid substance, granulovacuolar degeneration, and Hirano bodies.**

D. Myasthenia Gravis results from autoantibodies against the nicotinic acetylcholine receptor on skeletal muscle. Thymic cells augment B-cell production of autoantibodies. The cardinal manifestation is fatigable weakness of the skeletal muscle. The extraocular muscles, including the levator palpebrae, are usually involved.

E. Lambert–Eaton Myasthenic Syndrome is caused by a presynaptic defect of acetylcholine release. It causes weakness in the limb muscles but not the bulbar muscles. Fifty percent of cases are associated with neoplasms (i.e., lung, breast, prostate). In these patients, muscle strength improves with use. In contrast, in patients with myasthenia gravis, muscle use results in muscle fatigue, autonomic dysfunction includes dry mouth, constipation, impotence, and urinary incontinence.

CASE 20-1

A 60-year-old man presents with progressive stiffness accompanied by difficulty walking and going down stairs. He has an expressionless face and a vacant, staring gaze. Examination reveals limited ocular motility in all directions. What is the most likely symptomatic therapy?

Relevant Physical Exam Findings

- Tremor at rest, with pill-rolling motion of the hand
- Rigidity observed when the patient's relaxed wrist is flexed and extended
- Bradykinesia

Diagnosis

- Parkinson disease is a progressive neurodegenerative disorder associated with a loss of dopaminergic nigrostriatal neurons. Often, patients are given levodopa combined with carbidopa. Nerve cells use levodopa to make dopamine to compensate for the loss of nigrostriatal neurons, whereas carbidopa delays the conversion of levodopa into dopamine until it reaches the brain.

Table of Cranial Nerves

Cranial Nerve	Type	Origin	Function	Course
I–Olfactory	SVA	Bipolar olfactory (olfactory epithelium in roof of nasal cavity)	Smell (olfaction)	Central axons project to the olfactory bulb via the cribriform plate of the ethmoid bone.
II–Optic	SSA	Retinal ganglion cells	Vision	Central axons converge at the optic disk and form the optic nerve, which enters the skull via the optic canal. Optic nerve axons terminate in the lateral geniculate bodies.
III–Oculomotor				
Parasympathetic	GVE	Accessory oculomotor (Edinger-Westphal) nucleus (rostral midbrain)	Sphincter pupillae; ciliaris	Axons exit the midbrain in the interpeduncular fossa, traverse the cavernous sinus, and enter the orbit via the superior orbital fissure.
Motor	GSE	Oculomotor nucleus (rostral midbrain)	Superior, inferior, and medial recti; inferior oblique; levator palpebrae	
IV–Trochlear	GSE	Trochlear nucleus (caudal midbrain)	Superior oblique	Axons decussate in superior medullary velum, exit posteriorly inferior to the inferior colliculi, encircle the midbrain, traverse the cavernous sinus, and enter the orbit via the superior orbital fissure.
V–Trigeminal				
Motor	SVE	Motor nucleus CN V (midpons)	Muscles of mastication mylohyoid, anterior bell of the digastric, tensor palati and tensor tympani	Ophthalmic nerve exits via the superior orbital fissure; maxillary nerve exits via the foramen rotundum; mandibular nerve exits via the foramen ovale; ophthalmic and maxillary nerves traverse the cavernous sinus; GSA fibers enter the spinal trigeminal tract of CN V.
Sensory	GSA	Trigeminal ganglion and mesencephalic nucleus CN V (rostral pons and midbrain)	Tactile, pain, and thermal sensation from the face; the oral and nasal cavities; and the supratentorial dura	

(continued)

Cranial Nerve	Type	Origin	Function	Course
VI–Abducent	GSE	Abducent nucleus (caudal pons)	Lateral rectus	Axons exit the pons from the inferior pontine sulcus, traverse the cavernous sinus, and enter the orbit via the superior orbital fissure.
VII–Facial				
Parasympathetic	GVE	Superior salivatory nucleus (caudal pons)	Lacrimal gland (via sphenopalatine ganglion); submandibular and sublingual glands (via submandibular ganglion)	Axons exit the pons in the cerebellar pontine angle and enter the internal auditory meatus; motor fibers traverse the facial canal of the temporal bone and exit via the stylomastoid foramen; taste fibers traverse the chorda tympani and lingual nerve; GSA fibers enter the spinal trigeminal tract of CN V; SVA fibers enter the tract.
Motor	SVE	Facial nucleus (caudal pons)	Muscles of facial expression, stapedius, posterior belly of digastric and stylohyoid	
Sensory	GSA	Geniculate ganglion (temporal bone)	Tactile sensation to skin of ear	
Sensory	SVA	Geniculate ganglion	Taste sensation from the anterior two-thirds of tongue (via chorda tympani)	
VIII–Vestibulocochlear				
Vestibular nerve	SSA	Vestibular ganglion (internal auditory meatus)	Equilibrium (innervates hair cells of semicircular ducts, saccule, and utricle)	Vestibular and cochlear nerves join in the internal auditory meatus and enter the brain stem in the cerebellopontine angle; vestibular nerve projects to the vestibular nuclei and the flocculonodular lobe of the cerebellum; cochlear nerve projects to the cochlear nuclei.
Cochlear nerve		Spinal ganglion (modiolus of temporal bone)	Hearing (innervates hair cells of the organ of Corti)	
IX–Glossopharyngeal				
Parasympathetic	GVE	Inferior salivatory nucleus (rostral medulla)	Parotid gland (via the otic ganglion)	Axons exit (motor) and enter (sensory) medulla from the postolivary sulcus; axons exit and enter the skull via jugular foramen; GSA fibers enter the spinal trigeminal tract of CN V; GVA and SVA fibers enter the solitary tract.
Motor	SVE	Nucleus ambiguus (rostral medulla)	Stylopharyngeus	
Sensory	GSA	Superior ganglion (jugular foramen)	Tactile sensation to external ear	
Sensory	GVA	Inferior (petrosal) ganglion (in jugular foramen)	Tactile sensation to posterior third of tongue, pharynx, middle ear, and auditory tube, input from carotid sinus and carotid body	
Sensory	SVA	Inferior (petrosal) ganglion (in jugular foramen)	Taste from posterior third of the tongue	

Cranial Nerve	Type	Origin	Function	Course
X–Vagal				
Parasympathetic	GVE	Dorsal nucleus of CN X (medulla)	Viscera of the thoracic and abdominal cavities to the left colic flexure [via terminal (mural) ganglia]	Axons exit (motor) and enter (sensory) medulla from the postolivary sulcus; axons exit and enter the skull via the jugular foramen; GSA fibers enter the spinal trigeminal tract of CN V; GVA and SVA fibers enter the solitary tract.
Motor	SVE	Nucleus ambiguus (midmedulla)	Muscles of the larynx and pharynx	
Sensory	GSA	Superior ganglion (jugular foramen)	Tactile sensation to the external ear	
Sensory	GVA	Inferior (nodose) ganglion (in jugular foramen)	Mucous membranes of the pharynx, larynx, esophagus, trachea, and thoracic and abdominal viscera to the left colic flexure	
Sensory	SVA	Inferior (nodose) ganglion (in jugular foramen)	Taste from the epiglottis	
XI–Accessory				
Motor (spinal)		Ventral horn neurons C1–C6	Sternocleidomastoid and trapezius muscles	Axons exit the spinal cord, ascend through the foramen magnum, and exit the skull via the jugular foramen.
XII–Hypoglossal		Hypoglossal nucleus (medulla)	Intrinsic and extrinsic muscles of the tongue (except the palatoglossus)	Axons exit from the preolivary sulcus of the medulla and exit the skull via the hypoglossal canal.

SVA, special visceral afferent; SSA, special somatic afferent; GVE, general visceral efferent; GSE, general somatic efferent; SVE, special visceral efferent; GSA, general somatic afferent; GVA, general visceral afferent; CN, cranial nerve.

APPENDIX II
Table of Common Neurological Disease States

Disease State	Characteristics
Acoustic neuroma	Derived from the Schwann cell sheath investing cranial nerve VIII; accounts for most tumors located in the cerebellopontine angle
Agnosia	Disorder of skilled movement; not due to paresis
Alzheimer's disease	Most common cause of dementia; anatomical pathology shows neurofibrillary tangles and senile plaques microscopically; cortical atrophy of the temporal lobe
Anencephaly	Neural tube defect in which the cerebrum and cerebellum are malformed while the hindbrain is intact
Aneurysm (cerebral)	Pathological localized dilatation in the wall of an artery
Anosmia	Inability to detect odors; may result from congenital defects (Kallman syndrome) or trauma
Anosognosia	Translates to "denial of illness" because patients denied their hemiplegia early after stroke
Anton syndrome	Form of cortical blindness in which the patient denies the visual impairment; results from damage to primary visual and visual association cortex of the occipital lobe
Aphasia	Language disorder resulting from stroke, trauma, or tumor of the dominant cerebral hemisphere; affects the patient's ability to produce and comprehend speech as well as the ability to hear and read words
Apraxia	Disorder of skilled movement in which the patient is not paralyzed but cannot perform basic activities; involves inferior parietal lobe and premotor cortex
Argyll-Robertson pupil	Small, irregular pupil that functions normally in accommodation but cannot react to light; often associated with neurosyphilis
Arnold-Chiari malformation	Congenital malformation of the hindbrain involving inferior displacement of the medulla, fourth ventricle, and cerebellum through foramen magnum
Astereognosis	Inability to recognize a familiar object when placed in the hand of a patient with eyes closed
Balint's syndrome	Characterized by poor visuomotor coordination and inability to understand visual objects; results from stroke of posterior cerebral artery
Benedikt's syndrome	Oculomotor palsy on the side of the lesion in the ventral midbrain (fascicular segment of cranial nerve III)
Cauda equina syndrome	Lower motor neuron lesion characterized by pain of the lower back and lower limb as well as bladder and bowel dysfunction; results from lesion of nerve roots of cauda equina
Chorea	Literally means "to dance;" patients cannot maintain a sustained posture; demonstrate "milkmaid's grip" and "harlequin's tongue"
Chromatolysis	Disintegration of Nissl substance in a neuronal cell body following damage to the axon
Conus medullaris syndrome	Characterized by both upper and lower motor neuron signs, including back and leg pain, paresthesias and weakness, perineal or saddle anesthesia, and urorectal dysfunction; often results from acute disc herniation
Dandy-Walker malformation	Congenital malformation characterized by underdevelopment of the cerebellar vermis, dilation of the fourth ventricle, and enlargement of the posterior cranial fossa; developmental delays, enlarged head circumference, and symptoms of hydrocephalus may be observed

Disease State	Characteristics
Duret's hemorrhage	Small punctate hemorrhages of the midbrain and pons resulting from arteriole stretching during the primary injury; may also result during transtentorial herniation as a secondary injury
Dysgraphia	Learning disability characterized by difficulty in expressing thoughts in writing; associated with extremely poor handwriting; results from head trauma
Dyskinesia	Involuntary movements often associated with extrapyramidal disorders such as Parkinson's disease
Dyslexia	Impairment in the ability to translate written visual images into meaningful language; common learning disability in children
Dysmetria	Lack of coordinated of movements of upper limb and eyes; characterized by under- or overshooting the intended position; closely related condition to intention tremor; may be associated with multiple sclerosis, in which it results from cerebellar lesions
Dysprosody	Characterized by alterations in rhythm and intonation of spoken words (prosody); associated with apraxia of speech; results from left frontal lesions adjacent to the Broca's area
Dystaxia	Literally means "no order"; involves loss of ability to grossly control skeletal muscles; characterized by dysphagia, dysarthria, and stiffness of movement
Foster Kennedy syndrome	Combination of papilledema in one eye and optic nerve atrophy in the other; characterized by visual loss in the atrophic eye; may also result from more distal remote ischemia or demyelination
Gerstmann's syndrome	Characterized by four signs, including writing disability (agraphia; dysgraphia), failure to understand arithmetic (acalculia; dyscalculia), inability to distinguish right from left, and an inability to identify fingers (finger agnosia)
Guillain-Barré syndrome	Peripheral neuropathy characterized by weakness affecting the lower extremities first, progressing superiorly to the arms and facial muscles; any sensory loss presents as loss of proprioception and areflexia
Hemianesthesia	Unilateral loss of sensation from the face; loss of pain and temperature sense on the contralateral side of the body
Hemianopia	Loss of half of the visual field
Hemiballism	Involuntary movements of the extremities, trunk, and mandible; associated with diseases of the basal nuclei (ganglia)
Hemiparesis	Unilatearl partial paralysis, resulting from lesions of the corticospinal tract
Herniation	High intracranial pressure shifts of the brain and brain stem relative to the falx cerebri, the tentorium cerebelli, and through foramen magnum
Hirschsprung's disease	Congenital disorder involving blockage of the colon due to dysfunction of smooth muscle contraction; results from abnormal neural crest cell migration into the myenteric plexus during embryonic development
Holoprosencephaly	Failure of the prosencephalon (forebrain) to develop
Horner's syndrome	Interruption of sympathetic innervation to the eye; characterized by three primary signs, including ptosis, miosis, and anhidrosis
Jugular foramen syndrome	Trauma to or tumor at the jugular foramen, with resultant paralysis of cranial nerves IX, X, and XI; often results from a basilar skull fracture
Kluver-Bucy syndrome	Lesion of medial temporal lobes and amygdala; characterized by oral and tactile exploratory behavior (inappropriate licking or touching in public); hypersexuality; flattened emotions (placidity)
Lambert-Eaton syndrome	Disorder of presynaptic neuromuscular transmission; impaired release of acetylcholine, resulting in proximal muscle weakness and abnormal tendon reflexes
Lateral medullary syndrome	Also known as Wallenberg's syndrome and posterior inferior cerebellar artery (PICA) syndrome; involves difficulty in swallowing and speaking; results from occlusion of PICA resulting in infarction of the lateral part of the medulla

(continued)

Disease State	Characteristics
Locked-in syndrome	Complete paralysis of all voluntary muscles of the body except the extraocular muscles; patients fully alert but cannot move; only movements of the eyes and blinking are possible; results from stroke in the pons
Lou Gehrig's disease [amyotrophic lateral sclerosis (ALS)]	Progressive degeneration of upper and lower motor neurons, resulting in hyperreflexia and spasticity (degeneration of the lateral corticospinal tracts) as well as weakness, atrophy, and fasciculations (due to muscle denervation)
Meningomyelocele	Cyst containing brain tissue, cerebrospinal fluid, and the meninges, protruding through a congenital defect in the skull; results from failure of the neural tube to close during gestation
Multiple sclerosis	Autoimmune disorder in which antibodies are created against proteins in the myelin sheath; results in inflammation of myelin and the nerves that it invests; causes scarring (sclerosis), which slows or blocks neurotransmission
Myasthenia gravis	Literally means "grave muscle"; chronic autoimmune neuromuscular disease characterized by weakness of the skeletal muscles of the body that worsens during periods of activity and improves after rest
Nystagmus	Involuntary rhythmic shaking or wobbling of the eyes; results from a pathological process that damages one or more components of the vestibular system, including the semicircular canals, otolithic organs, and vestibulocerebellum
Parinaud's syndrome	Bacterial infection of the eye, related to pinkeye, or conjunctivitis; tularemia may infect the eye by direct or indirect entry of the bacteria into the eye
Parkinson's disease	Disorder of the basal nuclei (ganglia) that results in resting tremor of a limb, slowness of movement (bradykinesia), rigidity of the limbs or trunk, and postural instability
Raynaud's disease	Vascular disease reducing blood flow to the extremities when exposed to environmental stimuli, including temperature changes or stress
Romberg sign	Results of a neurologic exam used to assess the posterior columns of the spinal cord involved in proprioception; a positive Romberg sign indicates sensory ataxia, whereas a negative Romberg sign suggests cerebellar ataxia
Subclavian steal syndrome	Occlusion of subclavian artery proximal to the origin of the vertebral artery; involves reversed blood flow in the vertebral artery; so named because it was thought that blood was stolen by the ipsilateral vertebral artery from the contralateral vertebral artery
Syringomelia	Cyst (syrinx) forms and expands within the spinal cord, destroying central tissue in the cord; results in pain, weakness, and stiffness in the trunk and limbs
Tabes dorsalis	Slow degeneration of the neurons in the posterior columns of the spinal cord; results in abnormal proprioceptive signals
Tic douloureux	Also known as trigeminal neuralgia; unilateral, severe, stabbing pain of the face, particularly jaw, cheek, or lip
Wallerian degeneration	Process of degeneration of the axons distal to a site of transection
Watershed infarct	Occurs at the junction of two nonanastomosing arterial systems; often between branches of the anterior and middle cerebral arteries
Wilson's disease	Also known as hepatolenticular degeneration; genetic disorder in which copper accumulates in the liver and basal nuclei (ganglia), specifically in the putamen and globus pallidus (lenticular nucleus)
Weber's syndrome	Also known as superior alternating hemiplegia; involves oculomotor nerve palsy and contralateral hemiparesis or hemiplegia; results from midbrain infarction as a result of occlusion of the posterior cerebral artery
Wernicke-Korsakoff syndrome	Neurologic disorder resulting from thiamine deficiency; usually caused by malnutrition, common in alcoholic patients; may present with vision changes, loss of muscle coordination, memory loss

GLOSSARY

abasia Inability to walk.

abulia Inability to perform voluntary actions or to make decisions; seen in bilateral frontal lobe disease.

accommodation Increase in thickness of the lens needed to focus a near object on the retina.

adenohypophysis Anterior lobe of the pituitary gland, derived from Rathke's pouch.

adenoma sebaceum Cutaneous lesion seen in tuberous sclerosis.

Adie pupil (Myotonic pupil) A tonic pupil, usually large, that constricts very slowly to light and convergence; generally unilateral and frequently occurs in young women with absent knee or ankle reflexes.

afferent pupil (Marcus Gunn pupil) A pupil that reacts sluggishly to direct light stimulation; caused by a lesion of the afferent pathway (e.g., multiple sclerosis involving the optic nerve).

agenesis Failure of a structure to develop (e.g., agenesis of the corpus callosum).

ageusia Loss of the sensation of taste (gustation).

agnosia Lack of the sensory-perceptional ability to recognize objects; visual, auditory, and tactile.

agraphesthesia Inability to recognize figures "written" on the skin.

agraphia Inability to write; seen in Gerstmann's syndrome.

akathisia (acathisia) Inability to remain in a sitting position; motor restlessness; may appear after the withdrawal of neuroleptic drugs.

akinesia Absence or loss of the power of voluntary motion; seen in Parkinson disease.

akinetic mutism State in which patient can move and speak but cannot be prompted to do so; due to bilateral occlusion of the anterior cerebral artery or midbrain lesions.

alar plate Division of the mantle zone that gives rise to sensory neurons; receives sensory input from spinal ganglia.

albuminocytologic dissociation Elevated cerebrospinal fluid (CSF) protein with a normal CSF cell count; seen in Guillain-Barré syndrome.

alexia Visual aphasia; word or text blindness; loss of the ability to grasp the meaning of written or printed words; seen in Gerstmann's syndrome.

Alzheimer disease Condition characterized pathologically by the presence of senile plaques, neurofibrillary tangles, granulovacuolar degeneration, Hirano bodies, and amyloid deposition; patients are demented with severe memory loss.

alternating hemianesthesia Ipsilateral facial anesthesia and a contralateral body anesthesia; results from a pontine or medullary lesion involving the spinal trigeminal tract and the spinothalamic tract.

alternating hemiparesis Ipsilateral cranial nerve palsy and a contralateral hemiparesis (e.g., alternating abducent hemiparesis).

altitudinal hemianopia Defect in which the upper or lower half of the visual field is lost.

amaurosis fugax Transient monocular blindness usually related to carotid artery stenosis or, less often, to embolism of retinal arterioles.

amnesia Disturbance or loss of memory; seen with bilateral medial temporal lobe lesions.

amusia Form of aphasia characterized by the loss of ability to express or recognize simple musical tones.

amyotrophic lateral sclerosis (ALS) A nonhereditary motor neuron disease affecting both upper and lower motor neurons; characterized by muscle weakness, fasciculations, fibrillations, and giant motor units on electromyography. There are no sensory deficits in ALS. It is also called *Lou Gehrig disease*.

amyotrophy Muscle wasting or atrophy.

analgesia Insensibility to painful stimuli.

anencephaly Failure of the cerebral and cerebellar hemispheres to develop; results from failure of the anterior neuropore to close.

anesthesia State characterized by the loss of sensation.

aneurysm Circumscribed dilation of an artery (e.g., berry aneurysm).

anhidrosis Absence of sweating; found in Horner syndrome.

anisocoria Pupils that are unequal in size; found in a third-nerve palsy and Horner's syndrome.

anomia Anomic aphasia; the inability to name objects; may result from a lesion of the angular gyrus.

anosmia Olfactory anesthesia; loss of the sense of smell.

anosognosia Ignorance of the presence of disease.

Anton syndrome (visual anosognosia) Lack of awareness of being cortically blind; bilateral occipital lesions affecting the visual association cortex.

aphasia Impaired or absent communication by speech, writing, or signs; loss of the capacity for spoken language.

aphonia Loss of the voice.

apparent enophthalmos Ptosis seen in Horner's syndrome that makes the eye appear as if it is sunk back into the orbit.

apraxia Disorder of voluntary movement; the inability to execute purposeful movements; the inability to properly use an object (e.g., a tool.)

aprosodia (aprosody) Absence of normal pitch, rhythm, and the variation of stress in speech.

area postrema Chemoreceptor zone in the medulla that responds to circulating emetic substances; it has no blood–brain barrier.

areflexia Absence of reflexes.

Argyll Robertson pupil Pupil that responds to convergence but not to light (near light dissociation); seen in neurosyphilis and lesions of the pineal region.

Arnold-Chiari malformation Characterized by herniation of the caudal cerebellar vermis and cerebellar tonsils through the foramen magnum; associated with lumbar myelomeningocele, dysgenesis of the corpus callosum, and obstructive hydrocephalus.

arrhinencephaly Characterized by agenesis of the olfactory bulbs; results from malformation of the forebrain; associated with trisomy 13–15 and holoprosencephaly.

ash-leaf spots Hypopigmented patches typically seen in tuberous sclerosis.

astasia-abasia Inability to stand or walk.

astatognosia Position agnosia; the inability to recognize the position or disposition of an extremity or digit in space.

astereognosis (stereoanesthesia) Tactile amnesia; the inability to judge the form of an object by touch.

asterixis Flapping tremor of the outstretched arms seen in hepatic encephalopathy and Wilson disease.

ataxia (incoordination) Inability to coordinate muscles during the execution of voluntary movement (e.g., cerebellar and posterior column ataxia).

athetosis Slow, writhing, involuntary, purposeless movements seen in Huntington disease (chorea).

atresia Absence of a normal opening(s) (e.g., atresia of the outlet foramina of the fourth ventricle, which results in Dandy-Walker syndrome).

atrophy Muscle wasting; seen in lower motor neuron (LMN) disease.

auditory agnosia Inability to interpret the significance of sound; seen in Wernicke's dysphasia/aphasia.

autotopagnosia (somatotopagnosia) Inability to recognize parts of the body; seen with parietal lobe lesions.

Babinski sign Extension of the great toe in response to plantar stimulation (S-I); indicates corticospinal (pyramidal) tract involvement.

Balint syndrome (optic ataxia) Condition characterized by a failure to direct oculomotor function in the exploration of space; failure to follow a moving object in all quadrants of the field once the eyes are fixed on the object.

ballism Dyskinesia resulting from damage to the subthalamic nucleus; consists in violent flailing and flinging of the contralateral extremities.

basal plate Division of the mantle zone that gives rise to lower motor neurons (LMNs).

Bell's palsy Idiopathic facial nerve paralysis.

Benedikt's syndrome Condition characterized by a lesion of the midbrain affecting the intraaxial oculomotor fibers, medial lemniscus, and cerebellothalamic fibers.

berry aneurysm Small, saccular dilation of a cerebral artery; ruptured berry aneurysms are the most common cause of nontraumatic subarachnoid hemorrhage.

blepharospasm Involuntary recurrent spasm of both eyelids; effective treatment is injections of botulinum toxin into the orbicularis oculi muscles.

blood–brain barrier Tight junctions (zonulae occludentes) of the capillary endothelial cells.

blood–cerebrospinal fluid (CSF) barrier Tight junctions (zonulae occludentes) of the choroid plexus.

bradykinesia Extreme slowness in movement; seen in Parkinson disease.

Broca's aphasia Difficulty in articulating or speaking language; found in the dominant inferior frontal gyrus; also called *expressive*, *anterior*, *motor*, or *nonfluent aphasia*.

bulbar palsy Progressive bulbar palsy; a lower motor neuron (LMN) paralysis affecting primarily the motor nuclei of the medulla; the prototypic disease is amyotrophic lateral sclerosis (ALS), characterized by dysphagia, dysarthria, and dysphonia.

caloric nystagmus Nystagmus induced by irrigating the external auditory meatus with either cold or warm water; remember COWS mnemonic: **c**old, **o**pposite, **w**arm, **s**ame.

cauda equina Sensory and motor nerve rootlets found below the vertebral level L-2; lesions of the cauda equina result in motor and sensory defects of the leg.

cerebral edema Abnormal accumulation of fluid in the brain; associated with volumetric enlargement of brain tissue and ventricles; may be vasogenic, cytotoxic, or both.

cerebral palsy Defect of motor power and coordination resulting from brain damage; the most common cause is hypoxia and asphyxia manifested during parturition.

Charcot-Bouchard aneurysm Miliary aneurysm; microaneurysm; rupture of this type of aneurysm is the most common cause of intraparenchymal hemorrhage; most commonly found in the basal nuclei.

Charcot-Marie-Tooth disease Most commonly inherited neuropathy affecting lower motor neurons (LMNs) and spinal ganglion cells; also called *peroneal muscular atrophy*.

cherry-red spot (macula) Seen in Tay-Sachs disease; resembles a normal-looking retina; the retinal ganglion cells surrounding the fovea are packed with lysosomes and no longer appear red.

chorea Irregular, spasmodic, purposeless, involuntary movements of the limbs and facial muscles; seen in Huntington disease.

choreiform Resembling chorea.

choreoathetosis Abnormal body movements of combined choreic and athetoid patterns.

chromatolysis Disintegration of Nissl substance following transection of an axon (axotomy).

clasp-knife spasticity Resistance that is felt initially and then fades like the opening of a pocketknife when a joint is moved briskly; seen with corticospinal lesions.

clonus Contractions and relaxations of a muscle (e.g., ankle or wrist clonus); seen with corticospinal tract lesions.

cog-wheel rigidity Rigidity characteristic of Parkinson disease. Bending a limb results in ratchetlike movements.

conduction aphasia Aphasia in which patient has relatively normal comprehension and spontaneous speech but difficulty with repetition; results from a lesion of the arcuate fasciculus, which interconnects the Broca and Wernicke areas.

confabulation Making bizarre and incorrect responses; seen in Wernicke-Korsakoff psychosis.

construction apraxia Inability to draw or construct geometric figures; frequently seen in nondominant parietal lobe lesions.

conus medullaris syndrome Condition characterized by paralytic bladder, fecal incon-tinence, impotence, and perianogenital sensory loss; involves segments S3–Co.

Corti organ (spiral organ) Structure containing hair cells responding to sounds that induce vibrations of the basilar membrane.

COWS (mnemonic) Cold, opposite, warm, same; cold water injected into the external auditory meatus results in nystagmus to the opposite side; warm water injected into the external auditory meatus results in nystagmus to the ipsilateral or same side.

Creutzfeldt-Jakob disease Rapidly progressing dementia, supposedly caused by an infectious prion; histologic picture is that of a spongiform encephalopathy; classic triad is dementia, myoclonic jerks, and typical electroencephalographic (EEG) findings; similar spongiform encephalopathies are scrapie (in sheep), kuru, as well as Gerstmann-Straüssler-Scheinker disease, which is characterized by cerebellar ataxia and dementia.

crocodile tears syndrome Lacrimation during eating; results from a facial nerve injury proximal to the geniculate ganglion; regenerating preganglionic salivatory fibers are misdirected to the pterygopalatine ganglion, which projects to the lacrimal gland.

cupulolithiasis Dislocation of the otoliths of the utricular macula that causes benign positional vertigo.

cycloplegia Paralysis of accommodation (CN III) (i.e., paralysis of the ciliary muscle).

Dandy-Walker malformation Characterized by congenital atresia of the foramina of Luschka and Magendie, hydrocephalus, posterior fossa cyst, and dilatation of the fourth ventricle; associated with agenesis of the corpus callosum.

decerebrate posture (rigidity) Posture in comatose patients in which the arms are overextended, the legs are extended, the hands are flexed, and the head is extended. The causal lesion is in the rostral midbrain.

decorticate posture (rigidity) Posture in comatose patients in which the arms are flexed and the legs are extended. The causal lesion (anoxia) involves both hemispheres.

dementia pugilistica (punch-drunk syndrome) Condition characterized by dysarthria, parkinsonism, and dementia. Ventricular enlargement and fenestration of the septum pellucidum are common; most common cause of death is subdural hematoma.

diabetes insipidus Condition characterized by excretion of large amounts of pale urine; results from inadequate output of the antidiuretic hormone (ADH) from the hypothalamus.

diplegia Paralysis of the corresponding parts on both sides of the body.

diplopia Double vision.

doll's eyes maneuver (oculocephalic reflex) Moving the head of a comatose patient with intact brainstem; results in a deviation of the eyes to the opposite direction.

Down syndrome Condition that results from a chromosomal abnormality (trisomy 21). Alzheimer disease is common in Down syndrome after the age of 40 years.

dressing apraxia Loss of the ability to dress oneself; frequently seen in nondominant parietal lobe lesions.

Duret's hemorrhages Midbrain and pontine hemorrhages due to transtentorial (uncal) herniation.

dysarthria Disturbance of articulation (e.g., vagal nerve paralysis).

dyscalculia Difficulty in performing calculations; seen in lesions of the dominant parietal lobule.

dysdiadochokinesia Inability to perform rapid, alternating movements (e.g., supination and pronation); seen in cerebellar disease.

dysesthesia Impairment of sensation; disagreeable sensation produced by normal stimulation.

dyskinesias Movement disorders attributed to pathologic states of the striatal (extrapyramidal) system. Movements are generally characterized as insuppressible, stereotyped, and automatic.

dysmetria Past pointing; a form of dystaxia seen in cerebellar disease.

dysnomia Dysnomic (nominal) aphasia; difficulty in naming objects or persons; seen with some degree in all aphasias.

dysphagia Difficulty in swallowing; dysaglutition.

dysphonia Difficulty in speaking; hoarseness.

dyspnea Difficulty in breathing.

dysprosodia (dysprosody) Difficulty of speech in producing or understanding the normal pitch, rhythm, and variation in stress. Lesions are found in the nondominant hemisphere.

dyssynergia Incoordination of motor acts; seen in cerebellar disease.

dystaxia Difficulty in coordinating voluntary muscle activity; seen in posterior column and cerebellar disease.

dystonia (torsion dystonia) Sustained involuntary contractions of agonists and antagonists (e.g., torticollis); may be caused by the use of neuroleptics.

dystrophy When applied to muscle disease, it implies abnormal development and genetic determination.

edrophonium (Tensilon) Diagnostic test for myasthenia gravis.

embolus Plug formed by a detached thrombus.

emetic Agent that causes vomiting; see area postrema.

encephalocele Result of herniation of meninges and brain tissue through an osseous defect in the cranial vault.

encephalopathy Any disease of the brain.

enophthalmos Recession of the globe (eyeball) with the orbit.

epicritic sensation Discriminative sensation; posterior column–medial lemniscus modalities.

epilepsy Chronic disorder characterized by paroxysmal brain dysfunction caused by excessive neuronal discharge (seizure); usually associated with some alteration of consciousness; may be associated with a reduction of γ-aminobutyric acid (GABA).

epiloia Tuberous sclerosis, a neurocutaneous disorder; characterized by dementia, seizures, and adenoma sebaceum.

epiphora Tear flow due to lower eyelid palsy (CN VII).

exencephaly Congenital condition in which the skull is defective with the brain exposed; seen in anencephaly.

extrapyramidal (motor) system Motor system including the striatum (caudate nucleus and putamen), globus pallidus, subthalamic nucleus, and substantia nigra; also called the *striatal (motor) system*.

facial apraxia Inability to perform facial movements on command.

fasciculations Visible twitching of muscle fibers seen in lower motor neuron (LMN) disease.

festination Acceleration of a shuffling gait seen in Parkinson disease.

fibrillations Nonvisible contractions of muscle fibers found in lower motor neuron (LMN) disease.

flaccid paralysis Complete loss of muscle power or tone resulting from lower motor neuron (LMN) disease.

folic acid deficiency Common cause of megaloblastic anemia; may also cause fetal neural tube defects (e.g., spina bifida).

gait apraxia Diminished capacity to walk or stand; frequently seen with bilateral frontal lobe disease.

gegenhalten Paratonia; a special type of resistance to passive stretching of muscles; seen with frontal lobe disease.

Gerstmann's syndrome Condition characterized by right-left confusion, finger agnosia, dysgraphia, and dyscalculia; results from a lesion of the dominant inferior parietal lobule.

glioma Tumor (neoplasm) derived from glial cells.

global aphasia Difficulty with comprehension, repetition, and speech.

graphesthesia Ability to recognize figures "written" on the skin.

hallucination False sensory perception with localizing value.

hematoma Localized mass of extravasated blood; a contained hemorrhage (e.g., subdural or epidural).

hemianhidrosis Absence of sweating on half of the body or face; seen in Horner's syndrome.

hemianopia Hemianopsia; loss of vision in one-half of the visual field of one or both eyes.

hemiballism Dyskinesia resulting from damage to the subthalamic nucleus; consists of violent flinging and flailing movements of the contralateral extremities.

hemiparesis Slight paralysis affecting one side of the body; seen in stroke involving the internal capsule.

hemiplegia Paralysis of one side of the body.

herniation Pressure-induced protrusion of brain tissue into an adjacent compartment; may be transtentorial (uncal), subfalcine (subfalcial), or transforaminal (tonsillar).

herpes simplex encephalitis Disorder characterized by headache, behavioral changes (memory), and seizures; the most common cause of encephalitis in the central nervous system. The temporal lobes are preferentially the target of hemorrhagic necrosis.

heteronymous Referring to noncorresponding halves or quadrants of the visual fields (e.g., binasal hemianopia).

hidrosis Sweating, perspiration, and diaphoresis.

Hirano bodies Eosinophilic, rodlike structures (inclusions) found in the hippocampus in Alzheimer disease.

holoprosencephaly Failure of the pros-encephalon to diverticulate and form two hemispheres.

homonymous Referring to corresponding halves or quadrants of the visual fields (e.g., left homonymous hemianopia).

Horner's syndrome Oculosympathetic paralysis consisting of miosis, hemianhidrosis, mild ptosis, and apparent enophthalmos.

hydranencephaly Condition in which the cerebral cortex and white matter are replaced by membranous sacs; believed to be the result of circulatory disease.

hydrocephalus Condition marked by excessive accumulation of cerebrospinal fluid (CSF) and dilated ventricles.

hygroma Collection of cerebrospinal fluid (CSF) in the subdural space.

hypacusis Hearing impairment.

hypalgesia Decreased sensibility to pain.

hyperacusis Abnormal acuteness of hearing; the result of a facial nerve paralysis (e.g., Bell's palsy).

hyperphagia Gluttony; overeating, as seen in hypothalamic lesions.

hyperpyrexia High fever, as seen in hypothalamic lesions.

hyperreflexia An exaggeration of muscle stretch reflexes (MSRs) as seen with upper motor neuron lesions (UMNs); a sign of spasticity.

hyperthermia Increased body temperature; seen with hypothalamic lesions.

hypertonia Increased muscle tone; seen with upper motor neuron (UMN) lesions.

hypesthesia (hypoesthesia) Diminished sensitivity to stimulation.

hypokinesia Diminished or slow movement; seen in Parkinson disease.

hypophysis Pituitary gland.

hypothermia Reduced body temperature; seen in hypothalamic lesions.

hypotonia Reduced muscle tone; seen in cerebellar disease.

ideational or sensory apraxia Characterized by the inability to formulate the ideational plan for executing the several components of a complex multistep act (e.g., patient cannot go through the steps of lighting a cigarette when asked to); occurs most frequently in diffuse cerebral degenerating disease (e.g., Alzheimer disease, multiinfarct dementia).

ideomotor or "classic" apraxia (ideokinetic apraxia) Inability to button one's clothes when asked; inability to comb one's hair when asked; inability to manipulate tools (e.g., hammer or screwdriver), although patient can explain their use; and inability to pantomime actions on request.

idiopathic Denoting a condition of an unknown cause (e.g., idiopathic Parkinson disease).

infarction Sudden insufficiency of blood supply caused by vascular occlusion (e.g., emboli or thrombi), resulting in tissue necrosis (death).

intention tremor Tremor that occurs when a voluntary movement is made; a cerebellar tremor.

internal ophthalmoplegia Paralysis of the iris and ciliary body caused by a lesion of the oculomotor nerve.

internuclear ophthalmoplegia (INO) Medial rectus palsy on attempted conjugate lateral gaze caused by a lesion of the medial longitudinal fasciculus (MLF).

intraaxial Refers to structures found within the neuraxis; within the brain or spinal cord.

ischemia Local anemia caused by mechanical obstruction of the blood supply.

junction scotoma Results from a lesion of decussating fibers from the inferior nasal retinal quadrant that loop into the posterior part of the contralateral optic nerve; in the contralateral upper temporal quadrant.

Kayser-Fleischer ring Visible deposition of copper in Descemet's membrane of the corneoscleral margin; seen in Wilson disease (hepatolenticular degeneration).

Kernig's sign Test method: subject lies on back with thigh flexed to a right angle, then tries to extend the leg. This movement is impossible with meningitis.

kinesthesia Sensory perception of movement, muscle sense; mediated by the posterior column–medial lemniscus system.

Klüver-Bucy syndrome Characterized by psychic blindness, hyperphagia, and hypersexuality; results from bilateral temporal lobe ablation including the amygdaloid nuclei.

labyrinthine hydrops Excess of endolymphatic fluid in the membranous labyrinth; cause of Ménière disease.

lacunae Small infarcts associated with hypertensive vascular disease.

Lambert-Eaton myasthenic syndrome Condition that results from a defect in presynaptic acetylcholine (ACh) release; 50% of patients have a malignancy (e.g., lung or breast tumor).

lead-pipe rigidity Rigidity characteristic of Parkinson disease.

Lewy bodies Eosinophilic, intracytoplasmic inclusions found in the neurons of the substantia nigra in Parkinson disease.

Lhermitte's sign Electriclike shocks extending down the spine caused by flexing the head; due to damage of the posterior columns.

lipofuscin (ceroid) Normal inclusion of many neurons and glial cells; increases as the brain ages.

Lish nodules Pigmented hamartomas of the iris seen in neurofibromatosis type 1.

lissencephaly (agyria) Results from failure of the germinal matrix neuroblasts to reach the cortical mantle and form the gyri. The surface of the brain remains smooth.

"locked-in" syndrome Results from infarction of the base of the pons. Infarcted structures include the corticobulbar and corticospinal tracts, leading to quadriplegia and paralysis of the lower cranial nerves; patients can communicate only by blinking or moving their eyes vertically.

locus ceruleus Pigmented (neuromelanin) nucleus found in the pons and midbrain; contains the largest collection of norepinephrinergic neurons in the brain.

macrographia (megalographia) Large hand-writing, seen in cerebellar disease.

magnetic gait Patient walks as if feet were stuck to the floor; seen in normal-pressure hydrocephalus (NPH).

medial longitudinal fasciculus (MLF) Fiber bundle found in the dorsomedial tegmentum of the brain stem just under the fourth ventricle; carries vestibular and ocular motor axons, which mediate vestibuloocular reflexes (e.g., nystagmus). Severance of this tract results in internuclear ophthalmoplegia (INO).

Mees lines Transverse lines on fingernails and toenails; due to arsenic poisoning.

megalencephaly Large brain weighing more than 1800 g.

meningocele Protrusion of the meninges of the brain or spinal cord through an osseous defect in the skull or vertebral canal.

meningoencephalocele Protrusion of the meninges and the brain through a defect in the occipital bone.

meroanencephaly Less severe form of anencephaly in which the brain is present in rudimentary form.

microencephaly (micrencephaly) A small brain weighing less than 900 g. The adult brain weighs approximately 1400 g.

micrographia Small handwriting, seen in Parkinson disease.

microgyria (polymicrogyria) Small gyri; cortical lamination pattern not normal; seen in the Arnold-Chiari syndrome.

Millard-Gubler syndrome Alternating abducent and facial hemiparesis; an ipsilateral sixth and seventh nerve palsy and a contralateral hemiparesis.

mimetic muscles Muscles of facial expression; innervated by facial nerve (CN VII).

miosis Constriction of the pupil; seen in Horner's syndrome.

Möbius syndrome Congenital oculofacial palsy; consists of a congenital facial diplegia (CN VII) and a convergent strabismus (CN VI).

mononeuritis multiplex Vasculitic inflammation of several different nerves (e.g., polyarteritis nodosa).

MPTP (1-methyl-4-phenyl-1,3,3,6-tetrahydropyridine) **poisoning** Results in the destruction of the dopaminergic neurons in the substantia nigra, thus resulting in parkinsonism.

multiinfarct dementia Dementia due to the cumulative effect of repetitive infarcts; strokes characterized by cortical sensory, pyramidal, and bulbar and cerebellar signs, which result in permanent damage; primarily seen in hypertensive patients.

multiple sclerosis Classic myelinoclastic disease in which the myelin sheath is destroyed, with the axon remaining intact; characterized by exacerbations and remissions, with paresthesias, double vision, ataxia, and incontinence; cerebrospinal fluid (CSF) findings include increased gamma globulin, increased beta globulin, presence of oligoclonal bands, and increased myelin basic protein.

muscular dystrophy X-linked myopathy characterized by progressive weakness, fiber necrosis, and loss of muscle cells; two most common types are Duchenne's and myotonic muscular dystrophy.

mydriasis Dilation of the pupil; seen in oculomotor paralysis.

myelopathy Disease of the spinal cord.

myeloschisis Cleft spinal cord resulting from failure of the neural folds to close or from failure of the posterior neuropore to close.

myoclonus Clonic spasm or twitching of a muscle or group of muscles, as seen in juvenile myoclonic epilepsy; composed of single jerks.

myopathy Disease of the muscle.

myotatic reflex Monosynaptic muscle stretch reflex (MSR).

neglect syndrome Results from a unilateral parietal lobe lesion; neglect of one-half of the body and of extracorporeal space; simultaneous stimulation results in extinction of one of the stimuli; loss of optokinetic nystagmus on one side.

Negri bodies Intracytoplasmic inclusions observed in rabies; commonly found in the hippocampus and cerebellum.

neuraxis Unpaired part of the central nervous system (CNS): spinal cord, rhombencephalon, and diencephalon.

neurilemma (neurolemma) Sheath of Schwann. Schwann cells (neurilemmal cells) produce the myelin sheath in the peripheral nervous system (PNS).

neurofibrillary tangles Abnormal double helical structures found in the neurons of Alzheimer's patients.

neurofibromatosis (von Recklinghausen disease) A neurocutaneous disorder. Neurofibromatosis type 1 consists predominantly of peripheral lesions (e.g., café au lait spots, neurofibromas, Lish nodules, schwannomas), whereas type 2 consists primarily of intracranial lesions (e.g., bilateral acoustic schwannomas and gliomas).

neurohypophysis Posterior lobe of the pituitary gland; derived from the downward extension of the hypothalamus, the infundibulum.

neuropathy Disorder of the nervous system.

Nissl bodies/substance Rough endoplasmic reticulum found in the nerve cell body and dendrites but not in the axon.

nociceptive Capable of appreciation or transmission of pain.

normal-pressure hydrocephalus Characterized by normal cerebrospinal fluid (CSF) pressure and the clinical triad dementia, gait dystaxia (magnetic gait), and urinary incontinence. Shunting is effective; mnemonic is **w**acky, **w**obbly, **w**et.

nucleus basalis of Meynert Contains the largest collection of cholinergic neurons in the brain; located in the forebrain between the anterior perforated substance and the globus pallidus; neurons degenerate in Alzheimer disease.

nystagmus To-and-fro oscillations of the eyeballs; named after the fast component; seen in vestibular and cerebellar disease.

obex Caudal apex of the rhomboid fossa; marks the beginning of the "open medulla."

Ondine curse Inability of patient to breathe while sleeping; results from damage to the respiratory centers of the medulla.

optokinetic nystagmus Nystagmus induced by looking at moving stimuli (targets); also called *railroad nystagmus*.

otitis media Infection of the middle ear, which may cause conduction deafness; may also cause Horner's syndrome.

otorrhea Discharge of cerebrospinal fluid (CSF) via the ear canal.

otosclerosis New bone formation in the middle ear resulting in fixation of the stapes; the most frequent cause of progressive conduction deafness.

palsy Paralysis; often used to connote partial paralysis or paresis.

papilledema Choked disk; edema of the optic disk; caused by increased intracranial pressure (e.g., tumor, epi- or subdural hematoma).

paracusis Impaired hearing; an auditory illusion or hallucination.

paralysis Loss of muscle power due to denervation; results from a lower motor neuron (LMN) lesion.

paraphrasia Paraphasia; a form of aphasia in which a person substitutes one word for another, resulting in unintelligible speech.

paraplegia Paralysis of both lower extremities.

paresis Partial or incomplete paralysis.

paresthesia Abnormal sensation such as tingling, pricking, or numbness; seen with posterior column disease (e.g., tabes dorsalis).

Parinaud's syndrome Lesion of the midbrain tegmentum resulting from pressure of a germinoma, a tumor of the pineal region. The patient has a paralysis of upward gaze.

Pick disease Dementia affecting primarily the frontal lobes; always spares the posterior one-third of the superior temporal gyrus; clinically indistinguishable from Alzheimer disease.

pill-rolling tremor Tremor at rest; seen in Parkinson disease.

planum temporale Auditory association cortex found posterior to the transverse gyri of Heschl on the inferior bank of the lateral sulcus; a part of Wernicke's area; larger on the left side in males.

poikilothermia Inability to thermoregulate; seen with lesions of the posterior hypothalamus.

polydipsia Frequent drinking; seen in lesions of the hypothalamus (diabetes insipidus).

polyuria Frequent micturition; seen with hypothalamic lesions (diabetes insipidus).

porencephaly Cerebral cavitation caused by localized agenesis of the cortical mantle; the cyst is lined with ependyma.

presbycusis (presbyacusia) Inability to perceive or discriminate sounds as part of the aging process; due to atrophy of the organ of Corti.

progressive supranuclear palsy Characterized by supranuclear ophthalmoplegia, primarily a downgaze paresis followed by paresis of other eye movements. As the disease progresses, the remainder of the motor cranial nerves becomes involved.

proprioception Reception of stimuli originating from muscles, tendons, and other internal tissues. Conscious proprioception is mediated by the dorsal posterior column–medial lemniscus system.

prosopagnosia Difficulty in recognizing familiar faces.

protopathic sensation Pain, temperature, and light (crude) touch sensation; the modalities mediated by the spinothalamic tracts.

pseudobulbar palsy (pseudobulbar supranuclear palsy) Upper motor neuron (UMN) syndrome resulting from bilateral lesions that interrupt the corticonuclear tracts. Symptoms include difficulties with articulation, mastication, and deglutition; results from repeated bilateral vascular lesions.

psychic blindness Type of visual agnosia seen in the Klüver-Bucy syndrome.

psychosis Severe mental thought disorder.

ptosis Drooping of the upper eyelid; seen in Horner's syndrome and oculomotor nerve paralysis (CN III).

pyramidal (motor) system Voluntary motor system consisting of upper motor neurons (UMNs) in the corticonuclear and corticospinal tracts.

quadrantanopia Loss of vision in one quadrant of the visual field in one or both eyes.

quadriplegia Tetraplegia; paralysis of all four limbs.

rachischisis Spondyloschisis; failure of the vertebral arches to develop and fuse and form the neural tube.

raphe nuclei Paramedian nuclei of the brain stem that contain serotoninergic (5-hydroxytryptamine) neurons.

Rathke's pouch Ectodermal outpocketing of the stomodeum; gives rise to the adenohypophysis (anterior lobe of the pituitary gland).

retrobulbar neuritis Optic neuritis frequently caused by the demyelinating disease multiple sclerosis.

rhinorrhea Leakage of cerebrospinal fluid (CSF) via the nose.

rigidity Increased muscle tone in both extensors and flexors; seen in Parkinson disease; cog-wheel rigidity and lead-pipe rigidity.

Romberg's sign On standing with feet together and closing eyes, subject loses balance; a sign of posterior column ataxia.

saccadic movement Quick jump of the eyes from one fixation point to another. Impaired saccades are seen in Huntington disease.

scanning speech (scanning dysarthria) Breaking up of words into syllables; typical of cerebellar disease and multiple sclerosis (e.g., I DID not GIVE any TOYS TO my son FOR CHRISTmas).

schizophrenia Psychosis characterized by a disorder in the thinking processes (e.g., delusions and hallucinations); associated with dopaminergic hyperactivity.

scotoma Blind spot in the visual field.

senile (neuritic) plaques Swollen dendrites and axons, neurofibrillary tangles, and a core of amyloid; found in Alzheimer disease.

shagreen spots Cutaneous lesions found in tuberous sclerosis.

shaken baby syndrome Three major physical findings: retinal hemorrhages, large head circumference, and bulging fontanelle. Eighty percent of the subdural hemorrhages are bilateral.

sialorrhea (ptyalism) Excess of saliva (e.g., drooling), seen in Parkinson disease.

simultanagnosia Inability to understand the meaning of an entire picture even though some parts may be recognized; the inability to perceive more than one stimulus at a time.

singultus Hiccups; frequently seen in the posterior inferior cerebellar artery (PICA) syndrome.

somatesthesia (somesthesia) Bodily sensations that include touch, pain, and temperature.

spasticity Increased muscle tone (hypertonia) and hyperreflexia [exaggerated muscle stretch reflexes (MSRs)]; seen in upper motor neuron (UMN) lesions.

spastic paresis Partial paralysis with hyperreflexia resulting from transection of the corticospinal tract.

spina bifida Neural tube defect with variants: spina bifida occulta, spina bifida with meningocele, spina bifida with meningomyelocele, and rachischisis; results from failure of the vertebral laminae to close in the midline.

status marmoratus Hypermyelination in the putamen and thalamus; results from perinatal asphyxia; clinically presents as double athetosis.

stereoanesthesia (astereognosis) Inability to judge the form of an object by touch.

"stiff-man syndrome" A myopathy characterized by progressive and permanent stiffness of the muscles of the back and neck and spreading to involve the proximal muscles of the extremities. The syndrome is caused by a disturbance of the inhibitory action of Renshaw cells in the spinal cord.

strabismus Lack of parallelism of the visual axes of the eyes; squint; heterotropia.

striae medullares (of the rhombencephalon) Fiber bundles that divide the rhomboid fossa into a rostral pontine part and a caudal medullary half.

stria medullaris (of the thalamus) Fiber bundle extending from the septal area to the habenular nuclei.

stria terminalis Semicircular fiber bundle extending from the amygdala to the hypothalamus and septal area.

Sturge-Weber syndrome Neurocutaneous congenital disorder including a port-wine stain (venous angioma) and calcified leptomeningeal angiomatoses (railroad track images seen on plain film); seizures occur in up to 90% of patients.

subclavian steal syndrome Occlusion of the subclavian artery, proximal to the vertebral artery, resulting in a shunting of blood down the vertebral and into the ipsilateral subclavian artery. Physical activity of the ipsilateral arm may cause signs of vertebrobasilar insufficiency (dizziness or vertigo).

sulcus limitans Groove separating the sensory alar plate from the motor basal plate; extends from the spinal cord to the mesencephalon.

sunset sign Downward look by eyes, in which the sclerae are above the irides and the upper eyelids are retracted; seen in congenital hydrocephalus and in progressive supranuclear palsy.

swinging flashlight sign Test to diagnose a relevant afferent pupil. Light shone into the afferent pupil results in a small change in pupil size bilaterally, and light shone into the normal pupil results in a decrease in pupil size in both eyes.

sympathetic apraxia Motor apraxia in the left hand; seen in lesions of the dominant frontal lobe.

syringomyelia Cavitation of the cervical spinal cord results in bilateral loss of pain and temperature sensation and wasting of the intrinsic muscles of the hands. Syringes may be found in the medulla (syringobulbia) and pons (syringopontia) and in Arnold-Chiari malformation.

tabes dorsalis Locomotor ataxia; progressive demyelination and sclerosis of the posterior columns and roots; seen in neurosyphilis.

tactile agnosia Inability to recognize objects by touch.

tardive dyskinesia Syndrome of repetitive, choreoathetoid movements frequently affecting the face; results from treatment with antipsychotic agents.

Tay-Sachs disease (GM_2 gangliosidosis) Best-known inherited metabolic disease of the central nervous system (CNS); characterized by motor seizures, dementia, and blindness; a cherry-red spot (macula) occurs in 90% of cases; caused by a deficiency of hexosaminidase A; affects Ashkenazi Jews.

tethered cord syndrome (filum terminale syndrome) Characterized by numbness of the legs and feet, foot drop, loss of bladder control, and impotence.

thrombus Clot in an artery that is formed from blood constituents; gives rise to an embolus.

tic douloureux Trigeminal neuralgia.

tinnitus Ringing in the ear(s); seen with irritative lesions of the cochlear nerve (e.g., acoustic neuroma).

titubation A head tremor in the anteroposterior direction, often accompanying midline cerebellar lesions; also a staggering gait.

tremor Involuntary, rhythmic, oscillatory movement.

tuberous sclerosis (Bourneville disease) Neurocutaneous disorder characterized by the trilogy of mental retardation, seizures, and adenoma sebaceum. Cutaneous lesions include periungual fibromas, shagreen patches, and ash-leaf spots.

uncinate fit Form of psychomotor epilepsy, including hallucinations of smell and taste; results from lesions of the parahippocampal gyrus (uncus).

upper motor neurons (UMNs) Cortical neurons that give rise to the corticospinal and corticonuclear tracts. Destruction of UMNs or their axons results in a spastic paresis. Some authorities include brain stem neurons that synapse on lower motor neurons (LMNs) (i.e., neurons from the red nucleus).

vertigo Sensation of whirling motion due to vestibular disease.

visual agnosia Inability to recognize objects by sight.

von Hippel-Lindau disease Disorder characterized by lesions of the retina and cerebellum; retinal and cerebellar hemangioblastomas. Non–central nervous system (CNS) lesions may include renal, epididymal, and pancreatic cysts, as well as renal carcinoma.

Wallenberg's syndrome Condition characterized by hoarseness, cerebellar ataxia, anesthesia of the ipsilateral face and contralateral body, and cranial nerve signs of dysarthria, dysphagia, dysphonia, vertigo, and nystagmus; results from infarction of the lateral medulla due to occlusion of the vertebral artery or its major branch, the posterior inferior cerebellar artery (PICA); Horner's syndrome is frequently found on the ipsilateral side.

Wallerian degeneration Anterograde degeneration of an axon and its myelin sheath after axonal transection.

Weber's syndrome Lesion of the midbrain basis pedunculi involving the root fibers of the oculomotor nerve and the corticobulbar and cortospinal tracts.

Werdnig-Hoffman syndrome (spinal muscular atrophy) Early childhood disease of the anterior horn cells [lower motor neuron (LMN) disease].

Wernicke's aphasia Difficulty in comprehending spoken language; also called *receptive*, *posterior*, *sensory*, or *fluent aphasia*.

witzelsucht Inappropriate facetiousness and silly joking; seen with frontal lobe lesions.